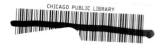

DATE			

Islamic
Medicine

Islamic Medicine

Muhammad Salim Khan

Routledge & Kegan Paul
London, Boston and Henley

First published in 1986
by Routledge & Kegan Paul plc

14 Leicester Square, London WC2H 7PH, England

9 Park Street, Boston, Mass. 02108, USA

Broadway House, Newtown Road,
Henley on Thames, Oxon RG9 1EN, England

Set in Palatino 11 on 13pt
by Columns of Reading
and printed in Great Britain
by Billing and Sons Ltd,
Worcester

Library of Congress Cataloging in Publication Data

British Library CIP Data also available
Khan, Muhammad Salim, 1951-
Islamic Medicine.

Includes bibliographies and index.
1. Medicine, arabic—history. I. Title.
/DNLM: 1. Medicine, arabic—history—Islam.
WZ 80.5.18 K45I/
R143.K54   1986   610'.917'671   85-25740

ISBN 0-7102-0329-2

To my mother
and
to my father, Dilbar Khan
for their love and affection

The Physician should be of a tender disposition, of wise and gentle nature, and more especially an acute observer, capable of benefiting everyone by accurate diagnoses; that is to say, by rapid deduction of the unknown from the known; and no physician can be of tender disposition if he fails to recognise the nobility of human being; nor of philosophical nature unless he knows logic, nor an acute observer unless he be strengthened by God's guidance.

Nidham-I-Arudi-I-Samarqandi

Contents

vii

Contents

Contents

Maps and diagrams

Maps

Diagrams

In the name of Allah, most merciful and compassionate

Preface

Today, we are living in a rapidly changing period of human history. Every aspect of human life is undergoing radical conceptual and practical changes and this includes the discipline of medicine. The monolithic and purely materialistic view of the world is being seriously questioned. There is growing concern with and alienation from our present destructive lifestyles which threaten the survival of humankind and their ecological and cultural environment. Consequently, there is a great searching, and a need for non-violent and ecologically safe alternatives. Within medicine, the concept of the whole person is once more replacing the fragmented view of the patient as a physio-chemical machine and a diagnostic jigsaw. There is increasing trust and confidence in natural and gentle methods of treatment. The importance of creative thought, balanced lifestyle and the healing forces within the individual are the important ingredients rather than strong chemical drugs.

It is in this context that this book on *Tibb-I-Islam* – Islamic medicine is presented. Aspects of the primordial wisdom, creative energy and rich tapestry of gentle and effective tradition, I hope and trust, will unfold before my readers.

Muhammad Salim Khan
Leicester England

Acknowledgments

I have been helped and supported by a number of individuals. In particular I wish to thank Dawood Relf, Abdul Rashid Skinner who helped my work when I most needed it and Peter Hopkins, who first suggested the idea of this book; *Hakim* Muhammad Nabi Khan for his guidance, hospitality and time; *Hakims* Lodhi, Dilpazeer, Niyazi and Noor Muhammad Hani for their suggestions and ideas, particularly Hani for his help on the principals of pulse diagnosis. J.D. Chapman also deserves my appreciation, for it is he who gave me the confidence in my early clinical days. Asghar Ali Abedi and ASAF Hussain for their encouragement and valuable advice. Ahmed, for his help with maps. Ann Humphries and Lailani Kennedy for their help and patience with correction and the typing of my almost illegible writing. Finally, a special thank-you and appreciation to Nasra, my wife, for her constant care and support whilst I was busy working on this book, almost oblivious to my family's needs.

CHAPTER 1

Historical background

We have sent among you an apostle (Muhammad, P.B.U.H) from among yourselves, rehearsing to you our signs, and instructing you in scripture and wisdom and in new knowledge.

The Qur'an 2:150

Health and medicine in pre-Islamic Arabia

Before considering the genesis and development of Islamic medicine, it would be useful to begin by enquiring into medical conditions before Islam. Pre-Islamic Arabia provides an interesting case study and comparative analysis with later Islamic civilisation. Consideration of the ecological and socio-cultural conditions in ancient Arabia would be an appropriate starting point. The Arabic term *Jazirat Al-Arab* – the Arabian peninsula, has come to be used for the whole of the Arabian peninsula which is situated on the east of the Red Sea and extends as far as the Modern Iranian Gulf.[1] The peninsula has considerable variation in climatic and ecological conditions which have influenced both the level and development of medicine.

1

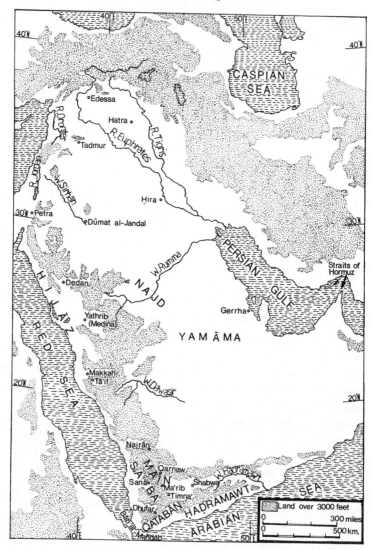

Pre-Islamic Arabia

Historical background

Within the Arabian peninsula is to be found one of the great desert regions of the world, covering an area of about 900,000 square miles. It is bordered in the west by the Red Sea, in the north by the Syrian Desert, in the south by the Arabian Sea and the Gulf of Aden and in the east and north-east by the Persian gulf, the Gulf of Oman and the Arabian Sea. There is almost always a breeze which changes seasonally to winds of gale force, cold or hot, which chill the body especially at night and roast it during the summer days. The summer heat is intense, with the interior of the peninsula being dry and tolerable. Coastal regions and some highlands, however, attain high humidity in summer with dew and fogs at night or in the early mornings.

The winters are invigoratingly cool with the coldest weather occurring at Taif, with several inches of snow and ice. Summer rains in Rub Al-Khalil accompany the monsoon winds from the Indian Ocean. Dominant winds blow from the Mediterranean, swinging to the east, south-east and south-west in a great arc. Two semi-annual windy seasons occur from December to January and from May to June. These are called *Shamals*, which try the patience of man and beast, are dry and transport huge loads of sand and dust, altering the shapes of sand dunes. Sharp drops in temperature are often followed by rain with wind velocities reaching gale force. On hot days the wind produces myriads of *Jinn* – dust devils and the ill-famed mirage.

The vegetation throughout the peninsula is varied. Plants are primarily xerophytic – those which grow in very dry conditions. After the spring rains long-buried seeds germinate and bloom. Date palm are grown in many oases in the desert, and across the peninsula.

3

Also found is rice, alfalfa, barley, wheat, citrus, melons, tomatoes, onions, and in higher regions peaches, grapes and pomegranates. Fish is in abundance in Al-Hijaz. Ancient Arabia was well known for its production of myrrh and frankincense, two important ingredients in the ancient civilizations of Egypt and Greece.[2]

Arabia has been inhabited by mankind since early times, and consequently Arabia has had many influences from different civilisations. Most of the ancient cultures have perished however.[3] The Arabs consider themselves to be descendants of Kahtan and Adnan. From these two ancestors arose numerous tribal units, forever splitting or confederating. Ancient Arabs lived as nomadic and semi-nomadic camel- and sheep-owning pastoralists in villages with agriculture. The cities have had merchant and religious classes. The Quraish of Makkah were an important group of tribes who controlled commerce and were in charge of the religious shrine of Kabbah. They organized two great trading caravans, one setting out in winter for Yemen, the other in summer for Syria. These were huge convoys bringing Oriental and African goods such as perfumes and silk. The visits of these caravans culminated in fairs with pilgrims at Makkah.

Although there have existed montheistic communities, pre-Islamic Arabia generally was polytheistic. Numerous deities were worshipped, the chief being Al-Lat, Al-Uzza and Manat.[4] Promiscuity was widespread and there were mass nude exhibitions and rituals in which both sexes took part.[5] The status and treatment of women was inhuman. Women had no right of inheritance and were considered a commodity. If a man died, the head of the clan would throw his gown over the widow as a gesture of acquisition which meant that the widow could not re-marry anyone except the owner of the gown. If he so wished he would marry her, or keep her in a state of bondage until she died.[6] Female-child infanticide was common. Newborn girls were buried alive or thrown to their premature deaths from high places.[7] This callous and inhuman practice left deep emotional trauma on members of the unfortunate families, including the father who had to perform the brutal act.[8] Tribal chauvanism was the hallmark of ancient Arabia. Tribal wars were a common occurrence fermented by interminable vendettas, with the killing of men and enslaving of children and women.[9]

The psychological implications of living in a society of ignorance and injustice were deep insecurity, excessive pride, guilt and dependence on alcohol. Alcohol for the pre-Islamic Arab was a psychological necessity. Life amidst oppression and stress created optimum conditions for the abuse of alcohol. It was so common that the Arabic word *Tajir*, which means merchant, became a synonym for the salesmen of *Khmar* – alcohol. The shops and bars of these merchants never closed during the day or night and were clearly distinguishable, being designated with special flags.[10] It is within this ecological and socio-economic environment that the level of health and medical knowledge of the pre-Islamic Arabs needs to be located. The general level of health was poor, and harsh climatic conditions were exacerbated by social injustice, poverty and ignorance. Thus it was fertile soil for the growth and proliferation of numerous diseases. The scarcity of a clean and adequate supply of fresh water was a permanent feature. The nutritional situation was poor, with a shortage of food and a monotonous diet. There were a number of endemic diseases – leprosy, malaria, tuberculosis, rickets, scurvy, numerous eye diseases and gastro-intestinal diseases.[11]

The pre-Islamic Arabs were familiar with the working of major internal organs, although only in general. Surgical knowledge and practices were limited to cauterisation, branding and cupping. The care of the sick was the responsibility of the women. There is no evidence of any oral or written treatise on any aspect of medicine. There was use of folk medicine, which has interesting connections with magic. It is also interesting to note that pre-Islamic Arabia had contacts with ancient Egypt, Greece, Persia and India, where medicine was highly developed, but there is no material to suggest that it was adopted or utilized by the ancient Arabs. This is particularly surprising in view of the fact that the ancient Arabs were well developed in their poetry.

Medicine in the early period of Islam

The beginning and development of Islamic concepts and practices of health are inextricably interwoven into the general body of Islam. The organic nature of Islam encompasses the core principles of Islamic health traditions. For an understanding of the historical or conceptual aspects of Islamic medicine reference to Islam itself has to be made. The earlier brief sketch of pre-Islamic Arabia provides a window onto the type of society at the time of Muhammad, peace be upon him. The proclamation by Muhammad, P.B.U.H., that he was the final messenger and prophet of Allah to mankind began with the *Wahy* – the revelation. Until this day Muhammad, P.B.U.H., had lived as a man, amongst pagan Arabs, working as a trader. The people of Makkah, where he was born and grew up knew him to be a reflective, gentle, kind and trustworthy man. The forty years that he spent amongst them led them to regard him as *Al-Ameen* – the trustworthy. The foundation of Muhammad's message was knowledge, based upon higher value. The first revelation placed knowledge, as its central focus, 'read in the name of Lord who created human being from clots of blood. Read! Your Lord is the most bounteous who has taught the use of the pen. Has taught human being what he did not know.'[12]

Thus the ignorance-based society of ancient Arabia was faced with Islam, which considered revealed knowledge to be its basis. The revelation continued to be a regular feature of the twenty-three years, and the repository of revealed knowledge became the Qur'an which, as a source of direct and pure knowledge, addressed itself to all facets of ancient Arabian belief and conduct. Whilst on one hand the Qur'an stressed the oneness of Allah and his powers, there was also the continued scrutiny of injustices and oppression. The Qur'an was clear and explicit in referring to these callous practices:

> When if one of them receive tiding of the birth of a female his face remains darkened, and he is wrath inwardly. He hides himself from the folks because of the evil of that whereof he has had tidings, (asking himself)! Shall he keep the child in contempt or bury it in the dust. Verily evil is their judgement.[13]

'And do not marry those women whom your fathers married . . . it was ever lewdness and abomination, an evil way.'[14]

7

Muhammad, P.B.U.H., continued his work for thirteen years in Makkah and within a decade he was able to attract most of the oppressed people, many of them slaves and poor. The small number of Muslims became increasingly victims to abuse, torture and killing. When the Quraish saw no success in their methods, they planned to kill Muhammad, P.B.U.H. News of this reached the Prophet and he decided to leave Makkah and migrate to the ancient city of Yathrib. (Later Yathrib was referred to as *Medina-Almunawra* – the illuminated city). It is from this event that Islamic dating begins which is known as the *Hijra*. It was in Medina that the Muslims became a community. As a community, as with other aspects of life and living, they began to develop a tradition of health and well-being that has continued to be practised in Muslim communities throughout the world. The ecological and climatic conditions in Medina were much more conducive to life and health than Makkah. Medina provided the conditions for the unfolding of *Shariha* – the Islamic way of life, of which medicine was an integral part. The Qur'an gave general guidelines and rules on nutrition, cleanliness, marital relations, child rearing, etc. As an example the Qur'an established the relationship between nutrition and behaviour. The concepts of *Halal* – lawful – and *Tayab* – wholesome – were linked to *Amal Salha* – constructive behaviour – and *Fisq* – destructive behaviour related to *Haram* – unlawful foods and beverages.

The messenger, P.B.U.H., laid great stress on the importance of sound health amongst his followers. He once said that: 'There are two gifts of which many men are cheated, health and leisure.'[15]

Muhammad, P.B.U.H., gave specific instructions on various aspects of healthcare and treated people

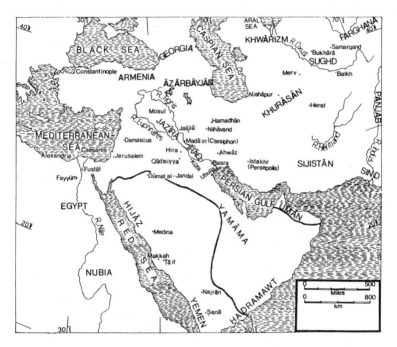

The time of the Prophet, P.B.U.H.

9

himself. He gave detailed information on specific diseases such as leprosy and infertility, with their causes and treatments. He prohibited certain types of treatments such as cauterisation and magic and introduced more appropriate ones. It was Muhammad, P.B.U.H., who told his companions not to embark upon treatment without adequate training. If any patient is harmed then the practitioner has to pay *Diya* – compensation.[16] The prophet Muhammad, P.B.U.H., provided the foundation for a medical tradition that considered a human being in its totality; the spiritual, the psychological and the physical within the context of a social milieu. The environment in Medina was one where ignorance and oppression was replaced with knowledge and justice. The level of health and well-being of the people of Medina was such that it appears miraculous. There was an enormous difference in the level of health between the pre-Islamic era to that in the new community of Muslims. A story from the period illustrates the health conditions:

> One of the kings of Persia sent to Muhammad, P.B.U.H., a learned physician. The physician remained in Arabia for one or two years but no one approached him or sought his treatment. At last he presented himself before the Prophet and complained: 'I have been sent to treat your companions but during all this time no one has asked me to carry out my duties in any respect whatever' to which the Prophet replied: 'It is the custom of these people not to eat until hunger overcomes them and to cease eating while there still remains a desire for food!' The physician answered: 'This is the reason for their perfect health,' kissed the ground in reverence and departed.[17]

Historical background

The period that followed the death of the Prophet, P.B.U.H., is referred to as *Khilafit-I-Rashida* – the right-guided rule. The Prophet had created a generation of men and women who became the torchbearers of knowledge and justice in the traditions introduced by him. It was during this period that the famous medical centre of Jundishapur became part of the Muslim lands and continued to flourish.[8] Companions of the messenger, such as Umar and Ali had become masters of matters of health and medicine. The prophetic teachings were interpreted by these men. New cities were built according to health principles and Muslim forces and travellers were given specific instructions on the maintenance of complete health. The period was an unfolding of the efforts of the Prophet, P.B.U.H., which he continued during his entire life. This was the period of rapid expansion of the Muslim community, with emphasis on collective responses on matters of health and social care.

The Umayyad period

In the forty-first year of the Islamic calendar (661 AD) Muawiya, grandson of the Umaiyyh of the Quraish tribe took over political control. The period that followed is generally referred to as the Umayyad Era. The Umayyad rule lasted until AH132 (AD 750) in the east and AH872 (AD 1492) in the west. It was during the Umayyad period that translations of ancient medical works were begun. The Umayyad prince, Khalid Bin Yazid, grandson of Muawiya was instrumental in this work. Khalid had a passion for medicine and alchemy. It was he who instructed a group of Greek scholars in Egypt to translate Greek-Egyptian medical literature into Arabic. These were the first translations made in Islam from one language to another, Khalid himself worked on medicine.[19] It was during this period AH120-198, (AD 737-812) that the most celebrated physician and alchemist, Jabr Ibn Hayan lived, a student of the well-known Iman, Jaffar Sadiq.

Muawiya, who first appointed Ibn Uthal as his personal physician, which became the practice with Umayyad governors such as Hajjaj Ibn Yusuf. However it was Walid B. Abdal-Malik who in AH88 (AD 707) began a broad health care programme. Walid had homes built for the blind and lepers. He isolated the lepers from other patients and provided medical facilities. He also built a hospital and appointed physicians who provided healthcare to all citizens and travellers on a free basis.[20] This was the beginning of free medical care on a mass level, supported from government funds. Under the Umayyads the Hispanic-Muslim areas of Cordoba and Granada became centres of learning. Economic prosperity, political stability and an emphasis on knowledge and tolerance provided ideal conditions for development. The rich and diverse flora of Spain was also a contributing factor. The development of botanical medicine was very high in Muslim Spain. Physicians like Ibn Al-Baytar, born in Malaga in AH598 (AD 1197) spent his early life in Andalusia, identifying and working on different plants. He also wrote a commentary on Dioscordies. His original contribution was a monumental work *Kitab Al-Mughni fil-Adwiyat Al-Mufridh* – the independent treatise concerning simple medicaments, which dealt with some 1400 different items used in treatment. This work became an authorative contribution to Materia Medica. Other well-known physicians were Abu Bakr Ibn Samghun of Cordoba, philosopher and physician

Historical background

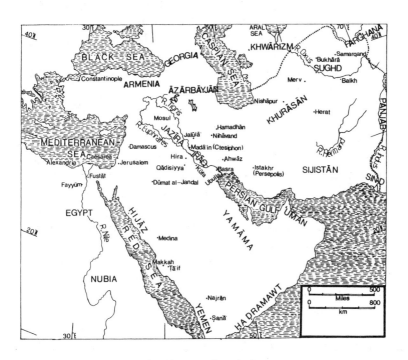

The Umayyad period

Ibn Bajjah, and Abul-Hassan Al-Andaluci also wrote extensively on plant remedies.[21]

Spain had a high level both of general medical practice and surgery. Abdul Qasim Al-Zahrawi, born at Madinat Al-Zahrai, near Cordoba in AH325 (AD 936) was one of the most capable surgeons. His systematic work *Kitab Al-Tasrif* – the Book of Concessions – was the definitive guide for surgeons. The text was accompanied with illustrations of each surgical instrument and was disseminated extensively.[22] In general medicine there were a number of scholar-practitioners in Spain writing and practising a wide range of therapies. Abu Marwan Ibn Zuhr composed *Kitab Al-Taysia Fil Mudawat Wal-Tadbir* – 'The Book Facilitating the Study of Therapy and Diet' – and *Kitab Al-Aghdiyah* – 'The Book of Diet'. Ibn Tufayl and Ibn Rushd were practising, and also contributed to medical research and literature.

The well-known Jewish philosopher and physician Abu Imran Musa Ibn Maymum, who later became personal physician to Salah Al-din Myamum, was an Andalusian and student of Ibn Rushid and Ibn Tufayl. Maymum wrote *Kitab Al-Fusul* – 'The Book of Aphorism' – and *Kitab Tadbir Al-Sihhah* – 'The Regime of Health' – as well as a number of other specific works. The development of medicine in its varied forms was a particularly important contribution of Umayyd-Muslim Spain. There were original contributions to surgery and internal medicine and the creation of new disciplines and specialities such as midwifery.

The Abbaside period

In AH 132 (AD 750) the house of Umaiyyah, the

Umayyads, were overthrown by Abdul Abbas Al-Abbas who was descended from Al-Abbas, the son of Abdul-Mutialib, a paternal uncle of Prophet Muhammad, P.B.U.H. For the next five centuries it was the Abbasides who dominated the socio-political life of the greater part of the Muslim world. There were major developments during the Abbaside period, particularly in medicine. The transfer of ancient medical knowledge which had begun with the Umayyads acquired greater momentum during the Abbaside period. The new impetus came about for a number of reasons. The most significant event was the founding of Baghdad in AH 186 (AD 754). It was Abu Jafar, known as al-Mansur, who founded the city of Baghdad on the banks of River Tigris in the most fertile area of Iraq. The site was also chosen for its ideal climate and absence of mosquitos. Al-Mansur had the city planned in such a manner as to be circular so that all the courtiers might be equidistant from the centre where the palace was built. The city was to be surrounded by a wall, pierced by four gates, each gate leading to Khorasan and Persia, to Basra and the South at Kufa and Arabia and to Syria and Byzantium.

The oldest suburb and the first to rise into great importance was that known as Karkh which lay to the south-west of the original walled city and was approached through the Kufa gate. Here was built the *Bimaristan* – the hospital which became the metropolitan hospital and the cradle of the Baghdad school of medicine. Here lectured and practised all the great physicians and surgeons of Baghdad from the time of Bukt Yishu, chief physicians from Jundishapur, to the most celebrated clinician and master of Arabic medicine, Razi. The hospital later was referred to as 'the old hospital'. The situation of the hospital must have been a delightful one for in front lay the great Karkhaya

Canal, a branch of the Isa Canal which joined the waters of the Euphrates to those of the Tigris.[23]

Al-Mansur, who was the second Abbaside ruler, suffered from dyspepsia throughout his life. Having tried his personal physician, Ibn Allahaj and others in vain, he turned to the physicians of the Jundishapur Medical School. Jundishapur was a flourishing centre of medical learning near the present city of Ahwaz in Iran. It was a cosmopolitan centre attracting scholars and physicians from Egypt, Syria, India, Greece and Persia. The chief physician at Jundishapur was Jurjis Ibn Bukht Yishu whose reputation as a skilled clinician had reached Al-Mansur. Bukht Yishu was invited to Baghdad, his treatment was successful and Al-Mansur appointed him his court physician at Baghdad. Bukht Yishu stayed in this capacity in Baghdad until near the time of his death when he asked Al-Mansur's permission to return to Jundishapur. This was granted and he died at Jundishapur in AH 149 (AD 769).[24]

The second phase of the development in medicine dated from the establishment of *Bayt Al-Hikmah* – the Royal Library – which became an important centre of translation of medical knowledge, based in Baghdad, the capital of the Abbasides. It was within *Bayt Al-Hikmah* that systematic and authentic translation and compilation was undertaken by competent scholars and physicians. There were separate sections dealing with literature from different languages. Jibrail Bukht Yishu, a descendant of Bukht Yishu migrated to Baghdad from Jundishapur. He established a medical practice in Baghdad, as well as writing and teaching. Yuhanna Ibn Masawayh whose father worked at Jundishapur also gained fame in Baghdad as an ophthalmologist. Ibn Masawayh became responsible for the translation of Greek texts and manuscripts into

Arabic. Hunayn Ibn Ishaq, a student of Ibn Masawayh was a prolific writer on medicine. He translated, from the Greek, Hippocrates, Galen and the Alexandrian summaries into Arabic. His original contribution was *Kitab Al-Ahsr Maqalat Fil Ayn* – 'Ten Dissertations on the Eye'. Thabat Ibn Qurrah compiled a work titled 'Treasury', which became a standard text on medicine. Ali Ibn Rabban Al Tabari wrote the well-known *Firdaws al-Hikmah* – 'The Paradise of Wisdom'. Al-Tabari used the medical contribution directly from Indian works. There were attractions in Abbaside Baghdad for physicians and scholars with many of them being invited to work for their patrons. An Indian physician, Mankha, was active in Baghdad translating Indian medical classics into Arabic.[25]

Within the two centuries under the Abbasides the medical heritage of ancient civilizations became accessible to Arabic scholars. In the *Bayt Al-Hikmah* scholars could work with all the necessary provisions and substantial income. The task of stocking the academy with new manuscripts became considerably facilitated due to the recent discovery of paper manufacture. Although paper was a Chinese discovery, it was introduced to the Muslim world when Samarqand was captured and the first paper manufacturing factory was established in Baghdad in AH 174 (AD 794).

The two centuries of Abbaside had made accessible to the Arab-speaking physicians the greater part of the classical medical heritage. The link in this important process was the new-found city of Baghdad. The next three centuries saw the synthesis and creation of new therapies. There were a number of original thinkers and practitioners whose contribution to Islamic medicine remains alive and pulsating. Muhammad Ibn Zakariyya Al-Razi was born in Rai in Persia. He studied music, alchemy and later medicine. He became responsible for the main hospital in Baghdad. He was a prolific medical scholar leaving many classical works such as the encyclopaedic *Al-Hawi* – 'Contents on Internal Medicine'. One of the most illustrious figures of this period was Abu Ali Ibn Sina, known as 'the Prince of Physicians'. Ibn Sina was born in AH 370 (AD 980) near Bukhra and travelled through Persia until his death in AH 428 (AH 1037).[26] Ibn Sina's most celebrated work is *Al-Qanun Fil-Tibb* – 'The Canon of Medicine'. Baghdad continued to be a centre of learning with a high level of medical practice and teaching. It was during the Abbaside period that the examination and licensing of physicians and surgeons was formally organized. However, the central role of Baghdad became less important after it was devastated by Halaku, grandson of Ghengis Khan in AH 640 (AD 1240).

Later works

After the devastation of Baghdad the history of Islamic medicine becomes much more diverse. Fortunately, before the invasion of Baghdad there had already been founded centres of medical learning in other parts of the Muslim world. The core concepts and practices of Islamic medicine continued to be common to various areas, although there were unique characteristics to each locality. Iran continued to be a source of medical inspiration for many years with a notable physician such as Sayyid Zayn Al-Din Ismail Al-Husayni Al-Jurjani who wrote *Dhakhira Y Khwarzam* – 'The Treasury of Medicine', dedicated to the King of Khwarzam. In Samarqand, Abu Hamid Muhammad

Al-Samarqandi composed *Kitab Al-Asbab Wal-Alamat* – 'The Book of Causes and Symptoms'. The Saffavid period continued with many new works on gynaecology. In Iran, it was from the reign of Nadir Shah onward that European medicine was introduced through the newly founded Centre Dar Al-funun in Tehran.[27]

In Egypt, under the Fatimids, Cairo became a centre of learning and started to attract competent physicians such as Maimondes who came over from Cordoba, Spain. Other reputable practitioners were Al-Latif Al-Baghdadi and Abd Al-Rahim Al-Dakhwar. The famous medical historian, Ibn Abi Usaybiah and the physician-surgeon Al-din Ibn Nafis were both Al-Dakhwar's students. Ibn Nafis was the first to explain accurately the minor circulation of the blood. He was born in Damascus in AH 607 (AD 1210) and died in AH 687 (AD 1288).[28]

Ottoman Turkey was also an important centre of Islamic medical knowledge. Similarly to other parts of the Muslim world, the Turks built numerous hospitals that were open to all people. The hospitals were generally regulated by trust deeds as welfare institutions. There were hospitals and medical schools built by the sultans which were both civil and military. A number of the later hospitals are still in active use in Turkey today. The language of medical instruction in Turkey was originally Arabic and was later changed to Turkish. Many of the well-known physicians wrote both in Arabic and Turkish. Initially, Turkish physicians travelled to Egypt but later Turkey became a centre for higher medical knowledge. The well known Turkish practitioners were many including Hakim Hae Pasa and Aydinoglu Umur Bey, known as Ibn Sina of Anatolia. It was a Turkish physician who first used small-pox vaccination in AH 1059 (AD 1679). It was during Sultan Mahmud II's reign AH 1209 (AD 1829) that European medicine came to be taught by Dr Bernard from Vienna, in French.[29]

The history of Islamic medicine in the Indo-Pakistan subcontinent is closely related to that of Iran. The primary language in Mogul India was Persian. Initially the language of medicine was Persian, although later Indian scholars transmitted medical literature into Urdu and also developed new methods. Indian physicians began to work closely with the Ayrvedic physicians which gave new impetus to Islamic medicine. India became the centre of medical learning with both traditions working very closely and at times in the same institutions and associations. India and Pakistan produced some of the most eminent physicians in later times. Akbar Arazani, author of *Tibb-I-Akbar* – 'The Great Medical Work' – was one of the last physicians of the Mogul period. Hakim Hafiz Muhammad Ajmal Khan of Delhi, known as *Masih-ul-Mulkh*, 'Healer of the Nation', one of his outstanding students and Hakim Muhammad Hussan known as *Shifla-Ul-Mulk*, 'Healer of the People', were the most celebrated custodians of traditional Islamic medicine in the twentieth century.[30]

CHAPTER 2

Philosophical conceptions of Islamic medicine

To begin with, we must recognise that the human organism is not an isolated entity, sufficient unto itself. Every individual is born, lives inseparably from the larger contexts of physical, social, political and spiritual influences. The laws governing the physical universe are not separate from those governing the functions of the living organism. So, we must begin by comprehending clearly the setting in which the human being is found, how it influences him, and in turn how he affects it. As with all things, the human organism was originally designed to function harmoniously and compatibly in the environment.

Vithoulkas

The problem of knowledge

The *Mesnavi* of Jalalu' din Rumi, a classic of wisdom contains a story called 'The disagreement as to the description and shape of the elephant'. It runs as follows:

The elephant was in a dark house. Some people had brought it for exhibition. In order to see it, many people were going, every one, into that darkness and, as seeing it with the eye was impossible, each

21

one was feeling it in the dark with the palm of his hand. The hand of one fell on the trunk: He said, 'This creature is like a water pipe.' The hand of another touched its ear: to him it appeared to be like a fan. Another handled its leg and said, 'I found the elephant shape to be like a pillar.' Another laid his hand on the back – he said, 'Truly this elephant is like a throne.' Similarly, when anyone heard a description of the elephant, he understood it only in respect of the part that he had touched. On account of the diverse place of view, their statements differed: One man entitled it 'Dal', another 'Alif'. If there had been a candle in each one's hand, the difference would have gone out of their words. The eye of sense perception is only like the palm of the hand: the palm hath not power to reach the whole of the elephant.

The genius of Rumi has penetrated to the centre of the problem of knowledge. Each hand fumbles over some part of the elephant, each proclaiming what they have discovered, and none is able to relate the part to the whole. The invention of instruments that render the senses a thousand or more times acute does not reduce the difficulties: if anything it increases them. Because of minute examination one is unable to listen to what is being said at the other end of the elephant. Even if it were possible to spare the time to study different disciplines or specialities, the search for knowledge has become so intense, so much data and observations have been accumulated, that no person can ever hope to know all that others have recorded. The prospect of synthesizing so much data seems an impossible task. It would seem that the very existence of an elephant has been forgotten. Consequently, the efforts are solely upon compilation of vast catalogues of observation on the trunk, legs or tail as the case may be.

This is the unsatisfactory state in which the whole body of knowledge finds itself. It is equally true of medical science: medicine studies the human being, which is an indivisible whole of such enormous complexity that it is impossible to grasp the truth about him. Modern medical science, therefore, has taken him to pieces in order to study each piece separately. The modern physician, called upon to deal with a sick human being, is confronted with a truly formidable task. What renders this task so difficult is the fact that the physician is unaware of what a normal human being is, still less a sick one. He has an acquaintance with the organs of a human being and has an idea as to how they work, but of the reality or nature of the human being himself, he is woefully and confessedly ignorant. Since the Renaissance in European society the fundamental conceptions of creation, life and human being have developed in mechanistic and materialistic paths to the exclusion of any higher values. In general, this view of the world has created fundamental problems, both technological and psychological, which have placed mankind on the edge of an abyss. In this context, the ethical and holistic perspective of the Islamic tradition of health provides hopeful insights.

Islam – an integrated unity

Any comprehensive tradition of medicine has a network of interdependent concepts and practices through which the origin, understanding, treatment and prevention of illness and maintenance of health is explained. Thus in reality there are close and intimately inseparable relations between the conception of a human being and health and disease.

Islam, as *Deen-I-Fithra* – the natural way of life, has its own paradigms of knowledge. The Islamic view of reality, provides a matrix in which central problems of knowledge are illuminated. Islam as a complete way of life has its own understanding of various aspects of life, including the maintenance of health and the alleviation of disease. For an understanding of the Islamic philosophy of medicine it is necessary to have a familiarity with the core values of Islam regarding the nature of creation, the position of humankind and the path of well-being.[1] Thus the health of an individual or a society can only be located within a context of Nature, society and man, as medicine is a facet of an integral view of reality. The essential outline of the philosophical tradition of Islamic healing is illuminated by the light of *Wahi* – revelation. The cosmos is the context and the human being is the subject. This philosophical perspective considers that genuine health and happiness is the natural state of existence. However, it can only be maintained or acquired by observing the fundamental laws of creation. It is in this respect that medicine needs to be located.

Tawhid – *The first principle and methodology of unification*

Islam as a universal principle lies in the nature of creation and comprehends a human being in its totality. The whole edifice of Islam is based on an understanding of *Tawhid* – a primordial concept of the oneness and unity of all creation. The ex-nihilo created universe is perceived through this principle. Unity is a world view and a mode of comprehension, a substratum upon which Islamic sciences in general, and medicine in particular, rests. Unity as a method perceives the cosmos as a dynamic, integrated and purposeful whole. It is a method of integration and means of becoming whole and realising the profound oneness of all creation. Every aspect of Islamic thought and action rotates around the doctrine of unity, which Islam seeks to realise in a human being in his inward and outward life. Every manifestation of human existence is organically related to the *Shadah* – witness. There is no deity except Allah, which is the most universal way of expressing unity. From this perspective the universe is viewed as a unity with varying levels of intelligence and will, in varying degrees. The universe is all the beings who populate the immensity of the skies, who constitute the regions of multiplicity which extend to the spheres, the stars, the elements, their products and humankind.

From this cosmological view the creation is divided into two relative and continuous aspects, influencing each other. *Gahib* – the unseen or hidden – and *Zahir* – the manifest. The manifest aspect of existence is accessible to sense perception and experience. These outer manifestations are *Ayat* – signs of the true essence. The outer and sensible manifestations are traces of primary and unseen reality. In this paradigm of knowledge there is an internal unity and integration between various levels of existence. Consequently, this philosophical and conceptual approach towards an understanding of reality has its own unique methodologies. One of the methods extensively employed by the scholars and practitioners is the symbolic language and analogy. The classical analogy of macrocosm and microcosm suitably illustrates the point.

In medical practice the analogy of the human being with the cosmos is used extensively:

> The body itself is like the earth, the bones like mountains, the brain like mines, the belly like the sea, the intestines like the rivers, the nerves like brooks, the flesh like dust and mud, the hair on the body like plants, the places where hair grows like fertile land and where there is no growth like saline soil. From its face to the feet the body is like a populated state, its back like a desolate region, its front like the east, back the west, right the south, left the north. Its breath is like the wind, words like thunder, sounds like thunderbolts. Its laughter like the light of noon, its tears like rain, its sadness like the darkness of night and its sleep like death. As its awakening is like life, the days of its childhood are like spring, youth like summer, maturity like autumn and old age like winter. Its motions and acts are like motions of stars and their rotation. Its birth and presence are like the rising of the stars and its death and absence like their meeting.[2]

The analogy is of profound significance, with practical implications in diagnosis and treatment. The micro-macro idea allows, through its profundity, the practitioner to penetrate beyond the physical realm. In the study of both nature and man, this idea provides a link in showing the unicity of creation, whilst demonstrating and enabling the inward relationship between them. Traditionally, the universe is macrocosm, or *Al-Insan-Al-Kabir* – 'the great man'. The universe is seen as one integrated body in all its spheres and gradation. It is also considered that the world has one *Nafs* – life force, whose powers run into all the organs and cells of its body, similar to a human being. In this respect analogies from the microcosms can illustrate an otherwise difficult concept. As an example, the relationship of the universal life force to the universe, described above, becomes vivid and easy to comprehend when compared to the human life force and the human body. Conversely, analogies from the universe can be used to explain the human being by correspondence drawn from the outer aspect. This is the broad context within which each individual is located. The multiferous influences from the different levels of the cosmos are an important consideration in the ability of man towards the maintenance of an equilibrium.

Human being – a microcosm

The creation of a human being occupies an important place in the philosophy of Islamic medicine. The origin, nature and purpose of humankind are important guidelines for the practitioner in enabling the patient towards health and well-being. The story of human creation is vividly illustrated:

Man did we create from a quintessence (of earth); then we placed him as (a drop of) sperm in a place of rest, firmly fixed; then we made the sperm into a clot of congealed blood; then of that clot made a (foetus) lump; then made out of that lump bones and clothed the bones with flesh; then we developed out of it another creature. So blessed be Allah, the best of creators.[3]

Like all of creation, human beings are created to live and function harmoniously within themselves and their surrounding. Each person individually, and mankind collectively, are endowed with an awareness and a consciousness. Creation is an *Ammna* – Trust – placed with mankind ideally and according to design, mankind has the potential to uplift and develop himself and the rest of creation, or degrade and abase himself and his environment. Thus, each person individually and human beings collectively, are simultaneously affecting and are affected by the wider environment. The purpose of human beings is *Ibadh* – serving and harmonising with the divine will. The outcome and result of *Ibadh* is an unconditional state of *Sakoon* – peace and tranquillity. The concept of *Ibadh* is a fundamental tenet of Islamic medical philosophy. Any evaluation of health has to take into account this central concept, as it is the key to an entire human integrity or dissipation at all level of the being, be they psycho-physio or psycho-spiritual. It is in this broad holistic perspective that the tradition of Islamic medicine is defined and located.

Tibb-I-Islami, Islamic medicine, is the body of practices that deal with the different states of *Insan*, the human being in health and disease. Its purpose is to maintain health and endeavour to restore it whenever lost. Health is a dynamic state in which all the functions are carried out in *Saheeha* – correct – and *Saleemah* – whole – manner.[4] This can be elaborated in that health is a dynamic condition of *Aitidal* – balance. It is a harmonious state of forces and elements composing the human being, as well as being external to him in conformity with the constructive principle in nature; each individual as a purposeful and integrated unity is always acting with innate intelligence to

28

maintain complete and dynamic condition of balance at different levels.

The Hakim – *a symbol of unity*

This holistic perspective and unity is reflected in the discipline of Islamic medicine. Indeed the principle of unity permeates and goes deep into the very structure of the cosmos and humanself. The practitioner of this medicine is a classical example. In this figure of the *Hakim* – sage and physician – one can see the unity of the sciences, as so many branches of a tree whose trunk is the wisdom embodied in the *Hakim*. The *Hakim* has always established the unity of the sciences in the minds of students by the very fact of his teaching all of the sciences as many different applications of the same fundamental principles. The Islamic teaching system as a whole and classification of the sciences which forms the matrix are themselves dependent upon this figure of the *Hakim*.[5]

CHAPTER 3

The psychological foundations

The question of the unity of the Divine Principle and the consequent unicity of nature is particularly important in Islam where the idea of unity (*al-tawhid*) overshadows all others and remains at every level of Islamic civilisation the most basic principle upon which all else depends.

Seyyed Hossein Nasr

The human being – an integrated whole

The paradigm of Islamic psychology is essentially derived from the core of Islamic traditions especially in the analysis of the *Nafs* – the self – and the means by which it can acquire its purpose, a state of unconditional tranquillity. *Qalb*, the heart, a non-material principle, is the essence of self and has predominant control of the life of an individual, by which reality is perceived and interpreted. The heart, from a traditional Islamic perspective, represents the whole human being in relation to *Al-Dunya* – the immediate condition and *Al-Akhira* – the approaching reality.[1] It is this essence which distinguishes human beings from all other created beings and constitutes the excellency which enables him to realise the truth. The heart is the point of union between *Jism*, the body, and *Ruh*, the spirit. In the Islamic order of creation the heart is the non-material centre of the human organism, that which registers and reflects conditions of consciousness. Changes can be initiated by external or an internal stimulus. It is on this plan that the essential functions such as the will, thinking and synthesis take place. Disturbance of these core functions constitutes a fundamental imbalance and disharmony within an individual. The heart is a centre of an organic whole of the psyche and the soma that guides, directs and controls the human organism towards the realisation of, and unification with, the truth.

The unity and diversity of Nafs – self

The most tranquil and balanced state of the self is *Al-Nafs Al-Mutmainna*.[2] This is the ideal to which the self can aspire and as a consequence of this state there is complete harmony within an individual in all realms of his functioning. The next state is one which is out of balance but has the ability and desire to be in tune; this condition is referred to as *Al-Nafs Lawwama*, the reproachful condition in which the self is active in gaining its lost balance.[3] The most unhealthy condition of the self is *Al-Nafs Al-Ammara*.[4] This is the condition of insensitivity and complete imbalance towards the destructive side of the spectrum. Thus we can see how the notion of tranquillity and balance is a central component in evaluation of the human condition and how it has far reaching consequence regarding the health of an individual.

The origin and functions of Rooh – vital force

The Muslim physicians consider man as a psycho-somatic unity endowed with a self-directing, purposeful *Rooh*, or vital force which issues from the left ventricle of the heart and enables activity, growth, forms and functions appropriate to the purpose of creation.[5] The vital force is a product of combination of *Latif* – subtle particles of the *Akhlaat* – the primary fluids and consequently the quantity and quality can be modified with appropriate changes in nutrition, medication and psycho-emotional factors. The vital force diffuses itself into the remotest parts of the organism and resembles the sun in luminosity. The vital force functions as an integrated totality in a systematic manner, according to laws of creation. An imbalance or disharmony within the vital force is the very beginning of disease, prior to any manifestations of pathology. Thus disease per se begins with the vital force, whilst functional or structural changes are secondary. The nature of the vital force is dynamic, penetrating and animating every organ and particle of human economy. The existence of vital force as an integral guiding principle within the human organism provides the Islamic science of healing with a logical, appealing and therapeutically useful entity whilst providing a conceptual basis for the unity of disease. We can examine, in some detail, the various physio-chemical functions of the vital force as it moves into different parts of the human organism. Although the vital force is one dynamic pulsating entity, in actual practice it has been divided into different parts on account of its functions, thus making it much more valuable in diagnosis and therapy.

Aspects of the vital force

That part of the vital force which issues forth from the left side of the heart is referred to as *Rooh Haiwania*, the vital faculty, due to its role as a vehicle for the maintenance of life within the human being. One of the major functions of the vital faculty is that it enables organs to receive life. The expansion and contraction of the vital force are subsumed by this faculty too.

Rooh Tabayya, the natural faculty, is of two types; that which is responsible for the preservation of the individual, centred in the liver, and that which is responsible for the preservation of the species, located in the testicles, or ovaries in the case of the female. The first type is essentially concerned with nutrition and growth while the second type is concerned with reproduction. For nutrition and growth to take place there are a number of processes that are necessary. Attraction, a process by which food is brought into the cells and tissues and is retained by retentive force until it has been digested by a digestive faculty. When the food is suitably digested it is assimilated and integrated into various cells and tissues.

Here *Quwat-ul-Mughaiyara* or the individuation faculty operates throughout the human body, functioning differently in the various organs according to their unique requirements. This need can be functional or structural. Each organ or system of the organism has an inherent natural faculty which enables it to make suitable changes in the nutrient. The process renders them one with each other in such aspects as colour and consistency. Conditions such as leucoderma, as an example, where absorption and assimilation are normal but wholeness is lacking, indicates defective individuation. Finally, the expulsive faculty is a process whereby non-nutritive matter, nutritive material in excess and material that has served its useful purpose and is no longer required is eliminated. It is useful to remember that waste matter is generally expelled through natural channels of elimination. However, when such outlets are not functioning properly, waste matter is diverted to an inferior organ, rather than a superior one, to a soft rather than a hard organ and to a less important organ than a more important one. This whole strategy of the vital force indicates inherent wisdom to safeguard the core of the person from disease.

For the successful perpetuation of the species there needs to be generative and formative faculties. The generative faculty is referred to as the faculty of primary individuation and is inherent within the semen. It is the first to appear in the development of the embryo. The generative faculty deals with the formation of male and female germinal fluids which have the ability to develop the various specialised cells, tissues and organs. The formative faculty gives shape, appearance and texture to the various parts, in conformity with the laws of creation.

That aspect of the vital force which is responsible for movement and sensation, and consists of cognition and conation is *Rooh Nafsania*, the nervous faculty, and is centred in the brain. Cognition is divided into two aspects: *Zahir*, the external or conscious, and *Ghaib*, the internal or unconscious. External cognition operates by means of five senses, namely vision, hearing, smell, taste and touch. Some consider touch to be a sense that has pain, temperature, smoothness or roughness, softness or hardness as its sub-divisions, thus considering eight senses in total. Conation is the process by which joints and organs are moved. This results from the transmission of impulses to muscles by means of corresponding nerves. Each muscle has its own mode of movement and activity, which is initiated by thinking, which is in turn subordinate to will.

Internal cognition or perception is a complex and intricate affair which has a number of processes. The composite sense is one that is located within the interior ventricle of the brain, and receives any image apprehended by the external senses and combines them into a coherent mental picture. The images formed are stored after their disappearance from the consciousness and this is carried out by *Quwa Mutafakkira*, thinking, which is different from imagination. When it serves *Al-Quwa-Al-Natqiya*, the rational mind, then it is termed thinking whereas when it serves *Wahm*, intuition, then it is referred to as imagination. There is a difference between thinking and imagination in that thinking can re-arrange the impressions and can produce not only images derived from perception but can occasionally add something more which is contrary to all perception, e.g. seeing an emerald mountain. Thinking is centred within the mid-ventricle of the brain.

Intuition is the process which gives an impetus to that which had no perceptual basis and is impelling and directive in many ways. Intuition can be a source of information protecting that which it believes to be important. Intuition's function is to discover the supra-sensual ideas and it is located within the extremity of the middle ventricle of the brain. Memory is located within the posterior ventricle of the brain, together with recall. Reasoning is a component of internal cognition. These various processes originating from external and internal sources are referred to the heart, which in the light of *Aql*, an apprehending light, deals with them according to the condition of the self. Thus we can begin to see that the idea of unity permeates throughout Islamic psychology with the heart as its pivotal point.

CHAPTER 4

Physiological concepts

All the four elements are seething in this world
None is at rest, neither earth nor fire nor water, nor air
Now earth takes the form of grass, on account of desire,
Now water becomes air, for the sake of this affinity
By way of unity, water becomes fire,
Fire also becomes air in this expanse, by reason of love.
The elements wander from place to place like pawn,
For the sake of kings love, not, like you, for past time.

Shamsi Tabriz

The fundamental concepts in Islamic Medicine have their basis within a traditional Islamic cosmology, a matrix for all the Islamic sciences. The manifestation of existence by being is a result of the polarisation of material prima into *quwa* – energy.[1] Muslim physicians and scientists subscribe to the theory that the highest level of organisation of the cosmos is not physical but one concerned with complex energy structures. The conception of the universe in terms of energy also extends to other organisms including human beings. This approach was developed by creating a spectrum for measuring the quality of energy. The four primary qualities of heat, cold, moisture and dryness are used as a qualitative aspect of measurement, heat and cold being active and moisture and dryness passive. The

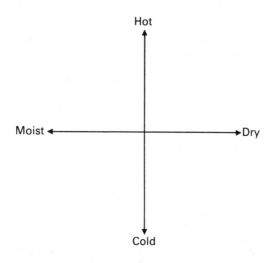

Figure 1   The polarisation of *quwa* – energy

concept of energy and its qualitative aspect were further developed into four basic universal symbols of the primary elements. The macrocosm, of which the human being constitutes the microcosm, is considered the resultant of the interplay of these four primeval elements which are united in an unvarying pattern.

Arrkan – *basic factors*

The *Arrkan* – the elements, is a symbolic reference to the actual fire, air, water and earth and not identical or per se.[2] The elements are simple bodies, primary components of all minerals, plants, animals and human beings. The various orders of being depend for their existence on a particular combination of the elements. The elements are subservient to the action of nature, a force present in all beings which directs and guides them.

> The earth is the warp and weft of the body.
> Heaven is man, and earth woman in character;
> whatever heaven sends it, earth cherishes,
> when earth lacks heat, heaven sends heat,
> when it lacks moisture and dew, heaven sends them.[3]

Earth is an element normally situated at the centre of all existence. In its nature it is at rest and all other elements naturally tend towards it, however great a distance away they might be. This is because of its intrinsic weight. Earth is cold and dry. In the scheme of creation it serves the purpose of rendering things firm, stable, lasting and heavy. It is by means of the earthly element that other parts are fixed and held together into a compacted form. Thus it is due to earth that the outward form is maintained. The vibration rate of the earth is slow. It is passive and receptive in nature like the female principle in creation.

Water is a simple substance whose position in nature is exterior to the orbit of earth and interior to that of air. This is due to its relative density. It is cold and moist. The purpose of water in the scheme of creation lies in the fact it lends itself to dispersion. Water provides, in the construction of things, the possibility of being moulded and shaped without permanency. Water being moist allows shapes to be readily fashioned. Water is the source of life as well as being essential to life.

Air is a simple substance, occupying the position

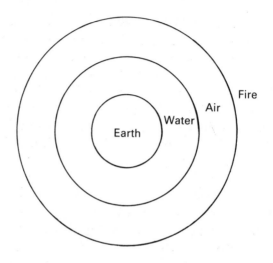

Figure 2   The relative position of the elements

above the sphere of water and beneath that of fire. This is due to its relative lightness. Air is hot and moist. In nature, in the process of creation, its purpose is to rarefy and render things finer, lighter and more delicate.

Fire is a simple substance, occupying a position in nature higher than that of the other three elements. Fire is hot and dry. The part fire plays in the creation of things is that it matures, refines and intermingles with all things. Its penetrative power enables it to permeate the substance of air. It thus subdues the coldness of earth and water and enables their integration into various compounds. Earth and water are required for the formation and the stability of the organs whereas the lighter elements, air and fire, are necessary for the production and the movement of the vital forces aiding the activity of the organs.

Akhlaat – *the humors*

Akhlaat is the biological application and extension of the elements. Muslim physicians conceived of the human body as a combination of *al-akhlaat al-arbah*, the four primary fluids, sometimes referred to as *banat al-arkan* – daughters of the elements. There are two types of fluids, normal and abnormal. Normal fluids are capable of being assimilated and integrated into tissue or energy, whilst abnormal fluids are unsuitable for assimilation and can be a source of imbalance and ill-health. There are four primary fluids: *Sauda, Bulghum, Dum* and *Safra* – black bile, phlegm, blood and bile, respectively. These four primary fluids in their normal state are responsible for the physiological, morphological and energy requirements of the body. Since the mucus membrane of the mouth is in direct continuity with the mucosa of the stomach, food begins to be changed and modified as soon as it comes into contact with the lining of the mouth. Saliva also promotes digestion, due to its innate activity. Within the stomach, digestion changes food into chyme, a juice-like fluid. Chyme is absorbed through the stomach and the small intestine into the liver. Liver works rapidly with this chyme maturing it and containing within it the four primary fluids. The main characteristics of the primary fluids are:

Sauda – as the Arabic word indicates is black bile; it is the sediment of normal blood. Black bile corresponds to the element Earth, being cold and dry in nature and possessing a retentive force. Its taste is

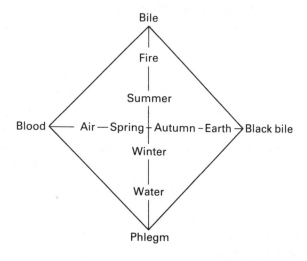

Figure 3   The relationship of seasons, elements and fluids

midway between sweetness and astringency. Black bile is associated with middle age and autumn and is active between 3 to 9 p.m. daily. The associative organs are the spleen, stomach and bones. Black bile is taken from the liver into the spleen and the blood. That bile which enters the blood is necessary for the nutrition of organs such as the bones. Within the blood itself, black bile makes it thick. That bile which enters the spleen is used by the spleen for nutrition and to purify the rest of the body of its excrementitious material and part of it is sent to the stomach. It renders the stomach firm, active, and induces hunger by its acidity. Abnormal black bile can be caused by excess heat or cold, inefficiency of the spleen, dietary indiscretions such as food containing thick, dry ingredients and negative emotional conditions. There are several varieties of abnormal black bile which are a source of ill health, particularly mental-emotional diseases.

Normal *bulghum* – phlegm is sweet, associated with the element water, and cold and moist in nature. It is dominant in old age, winter and during the night from 9 to 3 a.m. The related organs are the kidneys, the bladder and the brain, although it moves freely in the blood and joints. It possesses an expulsive force. Phlegm is different from the other fluids in that it can be converted into blood when necessary. It moistens the organs and joints to prevent dryness due to excess friction and heat. There are several varieties of abnormal phlegm and their main causal factors are lack of heat, working in water for long periods and an excess of phlegm-producing foods such as milk and cheese.

Normal *Dum* – blood is connected to the element Air, being hot and moist in nature. The associated organs are the lungs, blood and liver. Blood is active in childhood, spring and 3 to 9 in the morning. Normal blood is red, sweet and without smell. Blood possesses an attractive force. Its function is to provide nutrition to the organs and tissues. Abnormal blood can result due to excess of cold and heat, due to mixture with the other fluids, dietary mismanagement or emotional imbalance.

Normal *Safra*, bile, is yellow bile, corresponding to the element Fire, being hot and dry in nature. It is active in youth, summer and 9 to 3 during the day. Bile is light in weight, yellow in colour and possesses a digestive force. From the liver yellow bile is taken into the gall-bladder and the blood. The heart and the gall-bladder are the associative organs. That yellow bile which is taken into the blood makes the blood light and thin for easy passage through the capillaries. Yellow bile which enters the gall-bladder serves that organ and activates the intestines and rectum for defecation by peristaltic movements. Abnormal yellow bile can be due to its mixture with other fluids or due to a change of temperament. The causative factors can be excess heat, hot or sweet and greasy foods.

From these basic characteristic of the primary fluids we can begin to understand the relationship between the various factors. This simple and clear relationship begins to form a coherent picture indicating how closely and intimately interwoven are the relationship between diet, seasons, health and well-being.

Mizaj – *the temperament*

Mizaj – the temperament – is the dynamic state which results from the mutual interaction of the primary qualities inherent within the fluids. Every being is endowed with the most appropriate temperament for the purpose and conditions of its creation. Human beings possess the most suitable temperament for the conditions of life. Temperament is the inherent tendency or predisposition to respond along qualitatively predetermined individual characteristic patterns. Temperamental differences are the differences of response patterns to identical situations or stimuli. Each individual reacts according to an innate psycho-emotional pattern which makes that individual unique. The concept of temperament is a central clinical condition, significant in diagnosis and therapy. The essential sources of determining the temperament of an individual are morphological, physio-chemical and psychological signs: the practical ability to determine this must be developed over many years in a clinical setting. Since the primary qualities of the elements are four, the temperament of a newly organised body is a product of these qualities of heat, cold, dryness or moisture.

Theoretically, temperament is of two kinds: balanced, when the opposing qualities are quantitatively exactly equal and the balance is an average of these qualities and imbalanced when there is a dominance of any two of the four qualities. Imbalances of temperament can be further divided into eight varieties. In a simple imbalance of temperament the dominance may be an excess of heat or cold, without any excess of dryness or moisture, or an excess of dryness or moisture without any excess or heat or cold. However, simple imbalances do not last for long as they soon become compound. An imbalance in the direction of excessive heat will promptly lead to dryness and a change in the direction of cold will increase moisture.

Compound temperaments have dominances of two qualities such as hot and moist, hot and dry, cold and moist, and cold and dry. There is no coupling of heat with cold or dryness with moisture. The above-mentioned eight imbalances, four simple and four compound, have further gradations of each type into a further four degrees, depending on the strength of the imbalance. Thus in practice there can be multi-level gradation depending on the condition of the imbalance. The above imbalances can be of two kinds:

With morbid matter – temperament has become imbalanced due to an introduction of matter in the body such as excess phlegm or bile, etc.
Without morbid matter – these can arise per se and not

from any morbid matter, e.g. cold when exposed to snow.

There are other variations such as females being generally colder in temperament than men. They have a smaller build and have more relaxed tissues and muscles. Traditionally, the human life-span on earth is divided into four broad periods: growth which extends to twenty-eight years, maturity which lasts up to forty years, middle-age which extends up to sixty years, and finally senility. The period of growth is balanced in regard to heat but has an excess of moisture. During maturity there is a moderate excess of heat whilst in middle-age and old age there is an increasing proportion of cold.

The temperament of the organs

As mentioned earlier, each being as a whole is endowed with the most suitable temperament and likewise its individual parts and organs. In the case of man, each organ and member has also received the appropriate temperament requisite for its function, nature and conditions. There are some which are hot, others cold, others dry or moist. The degrees of dryness are as follows: hair is the dryest of the tissues as it is formed of smoky vapours solidified by the evaporations of moisture, the darker the hair, the dryer it is. Next are the bones, which are the hardest organs. They are slightly moister than hair as they are formed of blood with much black bile and absorb moisture from the muscles attached to them. This is the reason that a number of animals derive nutrition from them, whereas this is not the case with hair. Following in a descending order of dryness are cartilages, ligaments, tendons, membranes, arteries, veins, motor-nerves, the heart, sensory nerves and skin. The coldest component of the body is the phlegm, followed by hair, bones, cartilages, ligaments, tendons, membranes, nerves, the spinal cord, the brain, fat and skin. Phlegm contains the most moisture, followed by blood, fats, the brain, the spinal cord, breasts, testicles, lungs, liver, spleen, kidneys, muscles and skin. The hottest organ in the body is the vital force and heart, followed by blood, liver, muscles, spleen, kidneys, the walls of the arteries and skin. As a general principle, the organs rich in blood are hot and those poor in blood are cold in temperament. As it would be obvious from the gradation of various organs skin is the most balanced constituent, and in particular the skin of the terminal phalanges.

The temperament of medicines

Lo! The righteous shall drink of a cup
whereof the temperament is of camphor.[4]

In traditional Islamic medicine all living objects are categorised according to temperament based on the primary qualities of heat, cold, dryness or moisture. The temperament of articles of diet, items of aesthetic value, e.g. gem stones, and medicine are generally tested on healthy human beings, and these tests have rigorous standards upon which Materia Medica is built. There is a system of gradation based on the degree of change that a given substance can induce within a balanced individual. There is in fact an infinite number of gradations manifested in the equally infinite number of differences between substances, as was the case with temperament within individual persons. Thus, each substance has its unique temperament, modified by climate, habitat, etc. Compound medicines also have their own temperament which, in practice becomes much more difficult to assess. Thus, in actual therapy the physician needs to be conversant with the temperament of the articles of diet and medicine. In practice it takes many years to acquire and develop the practical art of analysis and diagnosis. We can begin to see the central importance in the evaluation of temperament in diagnosis and therapy. Specific details of signs of temperament will be discussed in a later chapter on diagnosis.

Aaza – *the organs*

The structure and functions of the human body form an extensive field of study requiring years of dedicated work. In this sub-section we wish to indicate an Islamic approach to the study of anatomy and physiology, rather than to supply extensive details. The unitary nature of knowledge in the Islamic sciences can be appreciated when studying human anatomy and physiology. According to the Islamic science of medicine, every cell, tissue and organ is created in a most perfect structure to fulfil its functions. The organs are primarily formed from the co-mingling of the fluids just as the fluids are derived from the primary elements. Every organ is endowed with an innate force for nutrition by which it absorbs, retains, assimilates and integrates its own nutrition and excretes the toxic and waste matter harmful to life and health. The constituents of the human body can be divided into simple and compound organs.

The *Aaza Mufrida* are those parts in which the visible and perceptible constituents convey the same name and definition as the whole. They are the bones, cartilage, nerves, tendons, ligaments, arteries and joints, membranes and flesh. These constituents are said to be homogeneous, as their particles or cells are of similar types.[5]

Aaza Murakiba are the organs of which the comprising parts, irrespective of size, differ in nature as well as name from the whole organ, e.g. hand. Thus, a part of the hand cannot be called a hand.

Compound organs are divided into a hierarchy of importance. The vital or principal organs are the heart, the brain, the liver and the generative organs. These are the centres of various functions and activities, absolutely necessary for the life of an individual and the species. The rest of the organs are auxiliary to the vital organs or are those which are instruments of their functions. The lungs are an example of the latter type. The following table indicates the two groups of auxiliary organs.

Vital organs	*Preparative organs*	*Auxiliary organs*
Heart	Lungs	Arteries
Brain	Stomach and liver	Nerves
Liver	Stomach	Veins
Testis/ovaries	Generative organs	Penis, ducts, uterus, etc.

We can begin to appreciate the unitary nature of anatomy and physiology with its gradation. Information and an understanding formulated in such a manner and methodology can be helpful to a physician in immediately evaluating the seriousness of any conditions upon taking up the case. Data organised in this systematic manner, based on natural laws can be of much more value in the analysis of a given individual's health-status than information derived from artificial classifications which ignore the order of creation. In this chapter a brief outline of the main physiological concepts used in traditional Islamic medicine has been described. The nature of the traditional health care approach in Islam is holistic and subtle, leading to a logical unity between the structure and function.

CHAPTER 5

Pathogenesis

This vital force is the one which is primarily deranged by
dynamic influences upon it of a morbific agent.

Hahnemann

Health, a dynamic condition of balance is the result of
an individual's ability to cope with internal and external
influences. The individual needs not only to create an
internal balance within himself but to adapt to social,
ecological and spiritual conditions.[1]

The *Hakims* over many centuries have delineated
essential factors that are fundamental to the maintenance of life and health. They are referred to as the
'six essential factors' and any imbalance in them
ultimately results in disease and premature death.[2]
They are:

– Ecological conditions
– Mental and emotional aspects
– Sleep and wakefulness
– Diet and nutrition
– Physiological movement and rest
– Retention and evacuation.

Ecological considerations

The multiplicity of influences of the universe upon any individual are numerous, from the most subtle, such as the spirit, to the most gross, such as the sun. Air is necessary for the maintenance of life and health and is an elementary constituent of human being. Man remains healthy as long as the air is balanced and free from pollution. Balanced air is free from fumes, chemicals, smoke and excess water vapour. Good quality air is that which is pure, clean, free from the vapours of ditches, ponds, waterlogged fields and foul gases from animal or vegetable remains. Good quality air is open to fresh breezes and comes from plains and high mountains. There are two essential functions of air:

 i) conditioning
 ii) purification of vital force.

Conditioning refers to the moderation of the temperament of the vital force. The vital force is moderated by air inhaled through the lungs and taken through the pores adjoining the arteries. The air that surrounds our bodies is generally much cooler than the normal temperature of the vital force. The contact and admixture of the vital force with balanced air prevents the vital force from becoming abnormal. Purification is the process whereby toxic vapours and substances are eliminated during expiration. The vital force is moderated by getting cooled during inspiration and purified during expiration.

Air has different effects depending upon its qualitative nature. Hot air is relaxing and produces dispersion. Moderate heat makes the complexion red, by drawing blood towards the surface. Excessively hot air can turn the complexion yellow and disperses the blood, producing excessive sweating and reducing the quantity of urine. It impairs the digestion and causes excessive thirst. Cold air makes the body firm, strengthens the digestion and increases the quantity of urine. Cold air hinders evacuation and prolongs stagnation. It separates water and diverts it towards the kidneys, leading to stools which are solid. Dry air makes the body thin and the skin dry and rough. Moist air softens the complexion and increases moisture.

Air can be the subject of changes which have implications for health. The changes can be normal or abnormal. Normal changes are the seasonal variations. Spring is considered the best season, as its temperament is suitable for the growth and preservation of life in general and the blood and vital force in particular. It is the time when trees sprout. Spring is out of all the seasons the most balanced and has the tendency to promote natural moisture and subtle heat. It promotes a rosy complexion and activates the humors but does not disperse them as in summer. Spring is a particularly suitable season for children and puberty. During spring the activation of the humors leads to certain diseases, particularly chronic diseases. Diseases of spring are nose bleeding, rupture of blood vessels, skin conditions such as abscesses and melancholia. Individuals with a phlegmatic temperament may suffer from such diseases as apoplexy and paralysis.

Summer tends to disperse the humors and the vital force, causing enfeeblement of the bodily functions. During summer there is a decrease in the quantity of blood and phlegm with consequent changes in the quality of the humors. Bile is increased during this season, giving a yellow tint to the complexion. During the latter part of summer there is a greater accumulation of black bile due to dispersion of light humors. Diseases of summer tend to be of short duration as the heat tends to mature and eliminate diseased matter. However, in individuals with low vitality, excess heat causes debility and can lead to death. Diseases of summer tend to be due to migration of the humors from the upper parts to the lower, such as diarrhoea. Febrile conditions are also common, as well as gangrene and infections of the eyes and ears.

Of all the seasons autumn is the one when disease is most prevalent. The reasons for this are that during autumn there is less blood as it is dissipated by the other humors, leaving excessive black bile. As this period starts to become cold there is a reduction of elimination and purification thus diverting humors inwards. Diseases of autumn are due to excess of black bile such as melancholia, cancer and joint pains. The expulsive faculty is weakened during autumn.

Winter aids digestion and is less prone to dispersion, but individuals who tend to have a sedentary life style, with excessive food intake during winter are predisposed to depressive conditions. It is a period which is cold and useful for reducing bile. Winter diseases are generally phlegmatic and the common cold and its effects are also prevalent at this time of the year. Winters which are particularly long and harsh are unfavourable to the old. There are also increased attacks of nervous disorders during this season.

Appropriate measures relevant to each season will be discussed in the chapter on treatment.

Mental and emotional factors

The core of an individual is the spirit which manifests itself through the mental and emotional channels. The different shades of emotions can be either positive, creative and life-enhancing or negative, destructive and death-promoting. Each emotion, depending on its quality and severity can influence the person, in particular the vital force. In general the movement of the vital force is outward and gradual in beneficial states, such as happiness and pleasure, whereas in conditions of sorrow, depression or fear the movement of the vital force is inward. Coma or at times death can occur due to sudden inward movement of the vital force, as in shock. Any prolonged movement towards negative aspects can predispose an individual towards serious mental-emotional and physical illness.

Sleep and wakefulness

Sleep is an important factor in the preservation and promotion of health. The quantity and quality of sleep is a significant cause of disease. Sleep removes fatigue and checks the flow of excretions due to the activities of the day. During sleep the innate heat is directed inwards, helping to promote digestion, growth and healing. It is due to the inward movement of the innate heat that the exterior of the sleeper becomes cold. The most beneficial sleep is that which is during the night, undisturbed, after a light, nutritious meal. Excess of sleep can predispose one to nervous diseases, dull the intellectual functions and cause accumulation of excess cold humours. Shortage of sleep is predisposed to create excess dryness with diseases such as mental confusion, itching and irritability. The effects of wakefulness are opposite to that of sleep.

Diet and nutrition

Amongst the various causes responsible for ill-health are articles of food and drink. Each separate item of food and drink, as well as in their different combination, has a specific effect on human health. The manner of eating, the psychological state of the person, the time of the day and year as well as the quantity and quality of food and drinks all need to be considered. In the Qur'an foods and drinks are divided into the two broad categories of *Halal* – lawful – and *Haram* – unlawful. The first category is further divided into a range of foods and drinks which are particularly health promoting and referred to as *Tayab* – wholesome. Each item of nutrition is further studied as to its qualitative aspect of being hot, cold, dry or moist. These four primary effects are then related to one of the four primary humors which may be blood, phlegm, bile or black bile. The quality and quantity of food and drinks is an essential tool in the maintenance and restoration of health. If we take water as an example, as an element it is taken as part of food and drinks, enabling food towards liquification, transportation and absorption. There are several types of water and that which is conducive to health should have the following qualities:

– it should be light in weight
– have a pleasant taste
– be easily turned hot or cold

– enable quick and easy cooking
– have no odour or colour
– it should quench the thirst.

An example of water with these qualities is the water from the Zam Zam spring in the valley of Hijaz in Makkah.[3] The best type of water is obtained from springs where the ground is pure and free from abnormal conditions, preferably from rocky mountains which are exposed to sun and fresh air. Rain water collected after a storm in an area where there are no external pollutants such as gases and chemicals is also health-promoting. However, rain water, due to its lightness, has a tendency to set up putrefactive changes. Water from snow or hail is generally impure. In hot climates or summer, ice and iced water can be used in moderation providing it is made from a pure supply of water. However, individuals suffering from conditions such as neuralgia or gastro-intestinal inflammation should refrain from iced drinks. Well water can be used, although it should be frequently lifted up from the well. Water from marshes should be avoided, as well as water containing heavy metals such as lead. Water infested with leeches and frogs is undesirable too. Specific waters rich in trace elements such as zinc or sulphur can be helpful in specific disease conditions, but must be used with caution.

Physiological movement and rest

Any form of activity whether prolonged or short, mild or vigorous produces heat in different degrees. However prolonged, activity which is mild produces the greater dispersion of humors. Different occupations produce their impact on health and cause specific diseases. An occupation such as that of washerwoman, undertaken over a long period results in a cold and moist condition, whereas a blacksmith can be predisposed towards excess heat and dryness. Rest is cooling and moistening, as there is little or no excitation of heat or inward accumulation of matter which subdues the heat.

Retention and evacuation

Any imbalance in retention and evacuation can be a cause towards disease. For maintenance of health there needs to be a balance between proper retention and elimination.[4] Imbalance in retention can occur when the expulsive force is weak or the retentive force is excessively strong. Improper digestion can lead to prolongation of obstruction of eliminative channels or thick and viscid matter. A crisis in illness can also cause retention. Diseases of excessive retention are moist and complex. Evacuation or loss of matter occurs when the conditions are contrary to those of retention. The diseases that occur due to excess evacuation are cold and debilitating.

CHAPTER 6

Diagnosis

The Physician should be of tender disposition, of wise and
gentle nature, and more especially an acute observer,
capable of benefiting everyone by accurate diagnoses; that
is to say, by rapid deduction of the unknown from the
known; and no physician can be of tender disposition if
he fails to recognise the nobility of human being; nor of
philosophical nature unless he knows logic, nor an acute
observer unless he be strengthened by God's guidance.
From Chahar Maqala of Samarqandi

Indications of health

Before considering disease and its symptoms it is
important to have an understanding of health. The
signs of a healthy person with a balanced temperament
are as follows:

- The complexion of an individual is pleasing with
  shades and colour that are normal to their respective
  biological environment
- Body build is medium, neither too lean nor too
  heavy

- Hair is not too profuse nor scanty
- Feel of the body is balanced in respect of heat, cold, moisture and dryness
- Sleep and wakefulness is moderate
- Movements are free and easy
- Intellectual functions and memory are good
- Habits and behaviour are balanced between timidity and assertiveness, anger and calm, leniency, humour, pride and humility
- Growth and repair is rapid whereas deterioration is slow
- Dreams are interesting and pleasing

The healthy person enjoys food, digests and assimilates normally and the excretory functions are regular.[1]

Classification of diseases

It has been emphasised that *Tibb* has an integrated approach towards health and disease in the context of spiritual, ecological and social environment. Over the centuries the practitioners of *Tibb* have evolved several classifications of disease. A disease is an imbalance that disturbs the harmony and balance which is natural to human beings. A disease may be described as medical, surgical, chronic or acute depending upon its nature or treatment. However, in any disease condition the unity of the person must not be forgotten, even though at any given moment the disturbance may be centred on a specific level or organ. There is a hierarchical division of diseases from above downward and from within outward, the most important level being above and within. This gradation can be depicted in diagrammatic form, the most central and

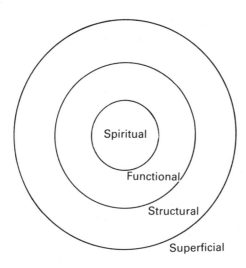

Figure 4 Hierarchical classification of diseases

crucial being the spiritual level and the least important being the peripheral.

The most important and highest level of an individual is the spiritual level. Disturbances on this level constitute the most fundamental imbalance. Imbalances on this level manifest themselves in the disturbance of the consciousness and mental functions. Conditions such as suicide, schizophrenia, delirium and total insanity are the result of disturbances on this plane.

Functional diseases are the disturbances that are manifested in imbalances of the temperament. These imbalances may be simple dominance of the active qualities of heat or cold or the passive qualities of dryness or moisture. However, simple imbalances are soon changed into compound imbalances and in this case a dominance of two qualities such as hot and moist, hot and dry, cold and moist or cold and dry comes into being. These imbalances of simple or compound type can arise either without any morbid matter or with morbid matter.

Structural diseases are diseases of the structure which may be of simple organs such as the bone or compound organs like the stomach. Structural disease may affect the size, number or form of an organ.

Superficial diseases are the diseases that manifest themselves on skin, hair, or other area of the complexion. Within the hierarchy this is the outermost aspect of an individual. However, the superficial diseases are the reflection of the inner working of the individual.

Signs of temperaments

The concept of temperament is of great importance in clinical practice, particularly in diagnosis. The notion of temperament is broad enough to encompass the structural and functional aspects of an individual.[2] The signs and indications of diagnosing the temperament are many. Here we will consider the major ones.

Body build is a helpful indicator of evaluating temperament of a person. A muscular body that is well-developed is a sign of heat and moisture, particularly when it is firm and solid. Poor muscular development with deficiency of fat is an indication of dryness. Fat, flabby and cold body is a reflection of cold temperament.

Complexion is also a sign which helps in the understanding of temperament. A pale or bluish tinge is cold and shows lack of blood. Yellow complexion points to excess of heat and bile. Dark complexion illustrates heat and dryness, whereas red or rosy colour shows heat and moisture.

As well as these general signs of temperaments there are more specific indications that help in diagnosing an individuals temperament:

Hot temperament: People of hot temperament have broad chest, well-developed body with good muscular growth, especially around the joints. This is due to the fact that heat promotes growth. These people are likely to have dark hair which is thick, profuse and grows rapidly. Their complexion may be dark or rosy. Their body is likely to feel hot when compared to that of a balanced person. The discharges or excretions of a person with a hot temperament are likely to have strong odours, high colour and full maturity. In individuals whose temperament is abnormally hot there may be additional signs and symptoms. They may feel uncomfortable in heat, excessive thirst, irritation and burning in the pit of the stomach, bitter taste in the mouth, intolerance of hot foods and drinks, craving of cold foods and drinks and excessive anger. All of these symptoms would get worse in summer and around midday.

Cold temperament: persons of cold temperaments have the opposite signs and symptoms than those of hot-tempered individuals. Cold hinders growth and maturity and these individuals are likely to have fat bodies that feel soft, flabby and cold to touch. They are also likely to have thin, scanty hair which is slow to grow. Their complexion is more inclined towards pale or white and chalky. The excretions or discharges such as urine and perspiration are inconsistent, sluggish and without strong odour. They are more likely to be sluggish and sleep excessively. In individuals whose temperament is abnormally cold there will be additional signs of weak digestion, absence of thirst, dislike of cold drinks and foods, craving of hot drinks and foods, colds and catarrhal discharges, laxity of joints, and all their symptoms becoming worse during winter and at night.

Moist temperament: people with moist temperaments are more likely to have similar symptoms to those of cold temperaments. However, in abnormally moist individuals there will be additional signs of excessive salivation, nasal discharges, diarrhoea, excessive sleep, puffiness of the body, especially under the lower eyelids, and intolerance of moist foods and habitat.

Dry temperament: Persons of dry temperaments have dryness and roughness of the skin with thin body, with prominence of joints and rapid growth of hair. In cases of abnormal dryness there may be additional indications such as insomnia, wasting, intolerance of dry foods, craving for moist foods and drinks, rapid absorption of light oils and worsening of symptoms in autumn.

Pulse

In the repository of wisdom and skills of Islamic medicine one of the most subtle and important tools for evaluation of health and disease is the pulse.[3] The pulse is the movement and contraction of the heart. The purpose of this movement is to condition the vital force. Each pulse-beat consists of two movements and two pauses. Thus there is expansion followed by pause with contraction accompanied by pause. Traditionally the pulse is felt by palpating the radial artery at the wrist. The reason for feeling the pulse at this point is that it is more accessible and can be examined without embarrassment to the patient, and it is in direct continuity with the heart. It is important that the pulse be examined when the person is calm without any stress, emotional or physical. The person being examined should be put at ease, and without full stomach. The person examining the pulse needs to be in a calm and balanced state of health. The necessary sensitivity and practical skill in examining the person has to be developed under supervision.

The study of pulse is complex and can be approached from different aspects. However, it is only possible to discuss the general principles governing the pulse. The physicians have laid down a number of features that provide valuable information helpful in the evaluation of health and the diagnosis of disease:

Size: the size of the pulse is noted by examining the degree of its expansion regarding the height, length and breadth. Thus in terms of the size the pulse has nine varieties which may be medium, long or short, medium, broad or narrow and medium, low or high. A pulse is considered long if it is longer than the pulse of the hypothetical absolute balance or the normal pulse of the person himself. A long pulse is an indication of excess heat and excess of activity. A short pulse is the opposite of the long one, indicating low heat and low activity. Medium pulse is a reflection of a balanced individual. The width of pulse gives an estimate of the amount of moisture. A wide pulse indicates excess moisture, whereas a narrow pulse is the opposite, with medium being the balanced state. The depth of the pulse is used to elicit the level of activity. A raised pulse points to a high level of activity with its opposite pointing to a contrary state, with the balanced level being the medium.

Temperature: the temperature of the pulse indicates the quality of the humours. A hot pulse indicates a hot quality humour, whereas cold pulse points to lack of heat. The moderate pulse is one showing balance.

Fullness: A full pulse reveals excess of humours. Empty or collapsed pulse is contrary in character and points to a deficiency of humours. A medium pulse is indicative of balance.

Duration of pulse: pulse is rapid or hurried when the period between the two beats is less than normal and is indicative of a fading vital force. The pulse is slow when this period is long, showing a strong vital force. A medium pulse is between the two extremes.

Constancy: A pulse may continue to be constant or vary in respect of the features illustrated above. A constant pulse is an indication of good health, whereas an irregular pulse points to weakness or disturbance. Irregular pulse can have numerous permutations too detailed to be mentioned in this work.

Strength or quality of impact: strength of the pulse gives indication of the quality of the vital force. The pulse which is felt by the pores of the fingers can be strong, which during expansion strikes forcibly against the practitioner's fingers. This variety of strong pulse indicates strong vital force. Weak or feeble pulse, the opposite of the strong type, is a pointer towards low vitality. A medium pulse is midway between the two types.

Speed or duration of cycle: speed of the pulse is an indication of a persons need for oxygen. The speed of the cycle of the pulse may be quick in which the duration of individual beats are shorter. This pulse is an indication of an individual's need for a greater amount of air. A medium type is between the two types, reflecting a balanced condition.

Consistency or elasticity: the elasticity of the pulse may be hard, pointing to excess dryness, or soft and easily compressible, reflecting excess moisture. A pulse of medium consistency is indicative of balanced moisture.

Urine

The excretion and discharges from specific organs and general body provide diagnostic indications. Urine as an example provides information about the functional states of the kidneys, digestive system, liver and spleen. However, it is important to consider the following conditions:

– urine should be collected in the morning before any drinks or foods have been eaten;
– no substance which can alter the colour of urine should have been taken, such as saffron;
– the individual giving the sample of urine should not have been unduly physically tired or mentally excited.[4]

Important points to be considered in using urine in diagnosis are colour, density, turbidity, sediment, quantity, froth and odour. Normal urine of an adult, healthy individual is of moderate density and pale yellow in colour. It is free from unpleasant smell, although it does have a smell. The sediments are not abnormal and there should be no irritation or burning.

The yellow colour has many shades such as orange, saffron, etc., and these different shades are an indication of overactivity and heat. Red, like yellow is also indicative of dominance of blood and heat. Any shade of green points to cold temperament as does white. Dark colouring points to excess of black bile and excessive combustion of humours.

Density of urine can be thin, medium or thick, each significant. Thick urine is a sign of defective maturation or elimination. Thick but clear urine is an indication of phlegm. Thin urine is due to incomplete maturation or weakness of kidneys, an obstruction or intake of fluids. Turbidity of urine is due to an admixture of *Reeh* – gaseous air with heavy particles. If urine is at first clear but becomes turbid on standing it indicates that the body is attempting to mature the morbid matter. Turbid urine which clears upon standing but leaves a deposit of coarse particles indicates successful maturation. Turbidity of urine can also be due to elimination of matter from liver, spleen or kidneys. In such cases, the findings need to be correlated with other diagnostic methods of pulse and stool.

Odour from a diseased person's urine is different from that of a healthy individual. Odourless urine is a sign of a cold temperament and immature humours. Foul-smelling urine can be a sign of ulceration in the kidneys or urinary tract. Sweet smelling urine indicates dominance of blood, whereas pungent smells point to excess of bile, acid or sour smell shows increased black bile.

The different types and amounts of sediment also provide diagnostic information. Any sample will have normal sediment and abnormal sediment such as pus. The quantity and quality of sediment is in chemical and physical aspects. In spite of adequate fluid intake, scanty urine is sign of low vitality. Passage of large quantity of urine with ease is a sign of improved vitality and recovery.

Stools

Occasionally conclusions may be derived from the condition of the stool of a person. Normal stools are compact, well-formed and passed without griping or irritation at regular periods. Usually almost odourless, free from froth and faintly yellow in colour.[5] In any consideration of stool analysis, the important factors are quantity, consistency, colour and sediment which may have been eliminated from the system through the stools. Quantity may be judged by taking into account the amount of food consumed. Large stools are indicative of dominance of humours, whereas scanty stools indicate a deficiency. The liquid stools point to indigestion, weakness of mesentric vessels or possible obstruction. Stools with froth, instead of being firm and compact, point to *Reeh* or excess of heat. Dry stools point to cold, polyuria or intake of dry foods.

Excess change in stool colour may be indicative of a disease process. Hyperfunction of bile can change the colour of the stools to excess yellow, whereas pale stool indicates lack of maturation. White stools can point to lack or obstruction of bile ducts. Black stool may point to excess of bile which may be indicative of serious illness. Pus and blood may also be a sign of serious illness. It is important to eliminate extraneous factors such as specific foods and medication which may alter the various colours or consistency of stool.

CHAPTER 7

Preventative aspects

All excess is against nature. Let your food, your drink,
your sleep and your sexual activity be all in moderation.

Hippocrates

Personal hygiene

One of the principal objects of the Islamic health care
tradition is to prevent suffering and disease prior to
any clinical manifestation. The entire life is guided and
directed towards wholesomeness and longevity with
the emphasis on prevention. Islam as an ethical and
holistic way of life deals with the spiritual and physical
aspects of an individual and the community. On the
spiritual and ethical levels teaching and practice
harmonize the inner consciousness with the outer
reality of creation. The clear and sublime perspective
focuses and liberates the individual from doubt,
confusion and subjugation to others and positively
helps to give purpose and meaning to life. This
wisdom is interwoven into daily living. A description
of the daily routine will give an insight into the
preventative dimension.

An individual is expected to get up early in the

morning *fajar* – before sunrise. After defecation and urination the person cleans both his hands with clean water and properly washes the anus and genital areas. The hands are then washed again, followed by the brushing of the teeth and gums. The teeth are cleansed with *miswak*, a traditional plant used from the early Islamic period for cleansing of teeth and oral hygiene.[1] The *miswak* cleanses the teeth as well as having antibacterial substances destroying the harmful germs in the mouth which cause infection and tooth decay. These wooden sticks are ecological and natural as well as being safe and economical. The mouth is washed three times with clean water. Next both nostrils are cleaned internally of mucus and externally of dust. The nose is washed with clean water using the left hand. Next the whole face is washed, beginning with the forehead, both eyes and ears. The cleansing of the face is followed by washing both arms from wrist to elbows with running water. After this moist hands are used to clean the head by running the hands from the top of the forehead to the back of the head. The tips of the fingers are used to clean the ears. This is completed by washing both feet up to the ankles starting from left to right, including the spaces between the toes and fingers. The *wudu* – physical cleansing – is started with the clear intention of focusing the attention on the inner aspect of purification. Each stage is sanctified by the recitation of specific passages from the Qu'ran. This purification is followed by *salah* – the most sublime spiritual commencement of the day. The *salah* can be offered collectively or individually.[2]

The person stands upright with his face towards the *qiblah*, directed at a point in the Grand Masjid in the city of Makkha. The consciousness is directed inwards. Both hands are raised gently and then the right hand is placed on the left, just below the navel. This is followed with passages of the Qu'ran. After the recitation and contemplation the hands are placed on the knees, followed by prostration on the floor. After prostration there is a period of sitting, accompanied by contemplation and recitation. This is a brief and general sketch of the external process of a profound and powerful form of integrated worship, offered at key intervals throughout the daily cycle. There are a number of stages within *salah* – sublime prayer – focusing the individual's inner self on particular aspects. The process culminates in supplication, the essence and marrow of the whole worship.[3]

Muslim physicians have developed the use of various modes of physical exercise that act as an effective prophylactic against various diseases, as well as strengthening the body. The wisdom of exercise is profound and far-sighted. It is an established fact that every organism requires food in order to survive and preserve health. However, even if the quality of the food is wholesome and easily assimilable by the body, it does leave a certain amount of waste. The eliminative organs try to eliminate the waste and toxins, but seldom succeed in clearing all of it. The waste that is left behind gradually accumulates with potential for disease. The waste and toxins can lead to a vitiation and disturbance of flow of energy and forces, abnormal changes in the general and specific organs, temperament, putrefaction and decay – particularly in the digestive tract – swelling and accumulation and abnormal growths.

It is these and other factors which dictate that steps need to be taken to eliminate waste and toxins. Exercise is one of the most effective and safe ways of eliminating waste products. The use of medication, unless in extreme and serious cases, is to be discouraged. Apart from the elimination of waste products, exercise stimulates the innate heat of the body, making the body stronger and lighter and building up the defences against harmful influences both external and internal. Exercise prevents the accumulation of wastes by dispersing and diverting it towards the eliminative organs and channels and assisting in expulsion of toxins. Thus with sound and regular exercise waste does not accumulate for long periods. The increase of innate heat stimulates the defences, burns out the insidious toxins and strengthens the joints and muscles. The exercise accelerates the absorption of nutrition by the tissues and organs. The organs are expanded and soften and the eliminative organs such as the skin pores are dilated. There is increased intake of oxygen, which in itself purifies and strengthens the entire body.

Exercise can be of two broad kinds: proper exercise which is carried out with the clear intention and purpose of benefiting, and exercise incidental to ordinary occupational or life activities. It is the former, proper exercise, which is the subject of our discussion and which wields maximum preventative benefits. The exercise can vary according to its mode, intensity and duration. It may be short or long, mild or strenuous, slow or rapid. It may also be rapid and strenuous or mild and slow. However, moderate exercise is the most suitable.

The strenuous exercises are many, such as boxing, wrestling, running, brisk walking, jumping, archery, fencing, horse-jumping, fighting one's shadow with a spear or sword. The general principle of these strenuous exercises is that they are strong and vigorous. Mild exercises are carriage-riding, slow camel-riding, cruising, swinging in a lying or sitting position, etc. Bathing in different waters and massage of various types are also forms of cleansing and exercise acting as preventative measures.

There is suitable exercise for every individual according to his or her specific constitution. The light or mild exercises are appropriate for persons debilitated from diseases such as fever, and who are unable to move about quickly, or cannot stand for long periods. Persons who have used purgatives or are suffering from respiratory conditions such as pleurisy are advised to take mild exercise. The elderly are also recommended these kind of exercises and the benefits and effects of them are relaxation and sleepiness and the dispersion of *reeh* – harmful gases. It helps in poor memory and certain cases of brain damage, stimulates the appetite and helps in conditions of mild depression. Similarly, riding in horse-drawn carriages has beneficial effects but is slightly more potent and may produce shaking of the body. Voyaging and cruising in small vessels close to the coastline is useful in certain speech disorders and skin diseases of dry types. Cruising in deep waters can be beneficial in certain emotional conditions, but there is generation of fear.

Youth and adult life, in general, is the time for strenuous exercise as well as when specific areas need to be strengthened. There are also exercises for individual organs which have particular benefits. For the improvement of eyesight, occasional gazing at water, green plants and minute objects intently, but without fixing the eyes for too long are some examples. Listening attentively to low-pitched sounds, occasionally interspersed with high pitched tones helps hearing. Thus each organ has a range of exercises which aid its function and structure. It is important to bear in mind that there are conditions in which exercise can be harmful and these need to be taken into consideration. The general rules are to protect the weak organs and the weak individual from strenuous exercise. In these cases exercise needs to be mild. There are some conditions such as varicose veins when movement of the part can be contra-indicated and in such conditions exercise should be given to the upper parts of the body and the legs rested. In diseases of the cerebral area, exercise of the head and neck needs to be taken with the advice of a physician. Similarly in the aged, and for pregnant women with diseases, it is advisable to consult a physician before taking systematic exercise.

There are some general rules for exercise of any type. The body needs to be in a state where food has been digested, but not empty. It should be taken at the point when the digestion is being replaced with assimilation. Before strenuous exercise there should be a warming-up period to stimulate the body gently. Massage before any exercise should be with a rough towel and after exercise with sweet oils such as almond. The bladder and bowels should be emptied before taking exercise. In hot climates or in summer it is advisable to exercise in the evening, or in cold climates or the winter at noon or in the morning. Exercise should be continued as long as colour is improving and the movement of limbs is easy and free, and sweat is evaporating. When these signs begin to disappear then exercise should be stopped. The end of exercise may be followed by a light massage with natural plant oils. Once a proper schedule of exercise is worked out it should be continued, unless there are reasons to the contrary.

There can be a number of complications from

exercise which need to be dealt with: there may be dryness, hydration, tightness, flaccidity or fatigue. Hydration can occur in individuals who live a sedentary and rich life, with frequent use of baths and much food. In these cases there should be dry massage and some recommendation of hard work. Dryness may be caused in an individual with a hot and dry temperament. In such cases rest and gentle massage with oils is the best solution. Flaccidity may be managed with a dry and vigorous massage and by use of an astringent oil. Stiffness is a frequent result of excess exercise, due to the drawing out of toxins from the tissues. Hot baths are helpful with light oil, moistening foods and rest. Fatigue is often experienced when there is excess or inappropriate exercise. Generally it disappears as soon as exercise is stopped. However, recuperative massage which directs the waste towards the skin, together with rest, helps.

Ghusl – bathing – is a necessary cleansing process which is used extensively in traditional health care. The *Hammams*, or baths of different kinds, are a normal feature in Muslim communities. There is extensive use of them by all sections of the community as preventative and curative aids. The particular benefits of bathing are induction of sleep, cleansing of the skin, removal of fatigue, dispersal of waste matters and drawing of blood toward the skin. Of course, indiscriminate and inappropriate use of bathing can be injurious. Excessive use may weaken the heart, produce nausea and fainting and disturb stagnant matter. General guidance with regard to bathing is to consider the season, the time of day, the condition of the stomach. Cold baths are most suitable in summer and in hot climates, whereas warm water should be used in winter and in cold regions. Cold baths should be avoided by weak, dyspeptic and catarrhal individuals.

Community health measures

Earlier in this chapter the Islamic approach to the spiritual and hygienic needs of an individual were illustrated. The balanced nature of the Islamic way of life is such that it deals with the community and has a collective dimension. Indeed, the term *ummah* used to describe Muslims means 'the community'. The emphasis on communal life is an Islamic approach. The individual can only develop within a harmonious integrated and well-knit community. From the early inception of the community in Medina, the Prophet, P.B.U.H., regulated and paid attention to health and hygiene. The cleanliness and promotion of specific and general matters of community health constitute an important aspect of Islamic medicine. The Prophet, P.B.U.H., dealt with issues of contagion and infection. About the plague he said:

> If you hear it has infected a certain area, stay away from it. But if it infects an area you happen to be in, do not move away from it to escape the disease.[4]

These and many other principles and practices were used in the formulation of community health policies and the organisation of environmental health. One of the central concepts and practices is the *taharah* – purification.[5] The Islamic classic medical texts deal with community health under separate studies referred to as *Hifz al-sihhah* – 'The Maintenance of Health'. The matters of sanitation, the quality and sources of water, the burial of the dead and other collective aspects of health are dealt with in considerable detail. Indeed there is advice to individuals attending collective prayers to refrain from eating raw onions and garlic and to use perfumes whilst attending community functions. It is the Islamic emphasis, when practiced and actualized, which enabled healthy and ecologically safe communities and wider environment.

Fasting – a specific institution of health promotion

Sawm – complete fasting – is one institution that combined the spiritual, physical, individual and community needs in a most harmonious way. The spiritual aspect of an individual is developed and enhanced in the most potent and sublime manner. *Taqwa* – God consciousness, discipline and empathy with the poor and needy – are the main emphasis behind fasting. Fasting as a devotional process and internal purification enables the person to transcend his gross physical needs. The deep cleansing process clears the mind and the internal organs and tissue. Biologically, fasting is an effective, natural process of detoxification and healing. Voluntary fasting is an intensely personal process. However, the manner of fasting in the Islamic tradition is a community affair.

The period of community regulated fasting is the month of Ramadan each year. The fact that the Islamic community uses a lunar calendar gives dynamism to the whole process. The months rotate according to the various seasons over the period. The four seasons of the year change from one season to another. Thus the individual enjoys the spiritual and physical benefits both preventative and curative at different periods. This timing itself indicates the natural and dynamic adaptability of Islamic health traditions to the needs of the individual and communities over time and space.

That fasting is a potent process must be taken into account and certain basic precautions should be noted. Children under the age of puberty are advised not to fast. Men and women who are old or have serious diseases need to consult a physician before embarking on the fast. Pregnant, or lactating women and also travellers need to be cautious and would be advised not to fast.[6]

CHAPTER 8

Principles of treatment

Within man there is a fleshy morsel, and when it is
corrupt the body is corrupt, and when it is sound the
body is sound. Truly it is the *qalb* – the heart.
                                    Muhammad, P.B.U.H.

Management of essential factors

Treatment in traditional Islamic medicine consists of a
number of different therapies selected and adapted to
both the general and the specific needs of an individual patient. The various levels of treatment are
management of essential factors, use of medicaments,
psycho-spiritual healing, manipulative measures and
surgical intervention. The management of essential
factors which was discussed in the chapter on patho-
genesis provides broad options capable of restoring
balance without the use of medicaments. Management
of the 'six essentials', as they are known sometimes,
consists of suitable modification. Food, one of these
factors, can be considered to illustrate this, using the
general principles for managing the quality and
quantity of food as a therapeutic measure. *Tibbi*,
nutrition, is based on the concept that for each food,

whether it is fruit, vegetable or meat, there is an energy, essence or state of quality that can be identified and formulated. The quality of the foods can be formulated by using the energy conceptual framework. This enables the physician to express the essence of food in a holistic manner and context.

In nutritional therapy, food can be withheld, increased, or given in moderate quantity, depending upon the needs and conditions of the individual patient and the nature of the disease. Food serves to provide energy and replaces the loss that results from the various activities of life and living. From an Islamic perspective there are the interconnections between food and the states of consciousness and emotional processes. In any disease there is an imbalance that also disturbs the various aspects of a person. The fact that an individual is regarded as one dynamic and integrated whole helps us to see the interconnections. Food is one of the most potent and yet safe instruments of establishing balance in a disturbed organism. Each individual ingredient of food is studied and understood in the holistic conceptual and empirical framework which was discussed in earlier chapters. The *Hakims* classify the range of foods on their qualitative basis of hot or cold and dry or moist. The qualitative nature of foods are part and parcel of common knowledge and folk traditions within Islamic communities. Traditionally, the selection of foods is based on season, age and needs of the individual. The therapeutic use of foods consists of using the qualitative understanding and quantity in a sensitive and controlled manner. A diet consisting mainly of fruit and vegetables is different in quality from, for example, half-boiled eggs and meats. Individuals with hot diseases such as fevers need essentially to use cooling vegetables of leafy types. Individuals with a good appetite but immature humors should be encouraged to change to a bulky diet. This will satisfy the appetite without adding to the quantity of the humors.

The quantity of food is generally reduced or stopped in acute diseases and sometimes in chronic conditions. In chronic conditions, the strength and vitality has been lost for considerable time and has to be maintained by the supply of food. In acute diseases, however, the crisis occurs quickly and it is expected that the strength will be sufficient to turn it into a healing crisis, culminating in health. The regulation of food at the critical stage of the disease, when the vital force is actively engaged in the struggle, requires a light diet. Indeed, the more acute the illness and the nearer the time of crisis, the lighter the food should be, unless there are any contra-indications.

Other factors in food management which are taken into consideration are rate of digestion and absorption of foods. Heavy and viscid foods such as beef are avoided in cases of stasis and obstruction. Assimilable and energy-giving foods such as honey are included when there is such a need in conditions following prolonged and protracted diseases. The psychological states and physiological conditions of an individual are also important considerations. The symbolic relationship of foods derived from cultural and religious sources must also be taken into account when planning any food therapy with an individual patient.

Treatment through a single remedy

In Islamic medicine there is a distinction between

Principles of treatment

Muffradat – single – and *Murakkabat* – compound medicaments.[1] The traditional use of individual substances in the treatment of various diseases still continues to be practised as the therapy of choice today. The range of substances used in the alleviation of suffering reflects the wide range of the richness that exists in Nature's treasury. Although remedies may be used from the mineral, plant and animal kingdoms, in practice, most remedies come from plant sources. In treatment, the principle that each human being is a reflection of all creation is followed by using a whole range of substances. Thus the analogy of micro-macro constitutes a biological reality and also has application in medical practice.[2] The use of the individual remedy is based on sound theoretical foundations and is supported by observations and experiments of countless generations of reputable physicians. Such empirical knowledge and wisdom, particularly in pharmocognosy is considerable and constitutes important skills in Islamic medical practice. The general emphasis in planning medicament therapy is to re-establish the lost balance within an individual patient with minimum intervention and change. The medicaments are used and selected after a meticulous and comprehensive life history, with particular reference to the medical aspects of an individual patient in the context of their family. The remedies are used in an active biological state rather than isolating a specific chemically or pharmacologically active element. The physician has to know each specific remedy in full detail:

– name of remedy
– identification and study of its natural habitat
– nature of the remedy

- its specific energy pattern
- physio-chemical actions
- indications of its uses in general and specific conditions
- specific relationship to organs
- duration of its action
- toxicity and contra-indications
- types of preparation
- dosage and administration, antidote

The modes of administration are many, depending on factors such as the nature of the disease, organ, etc. The general principle is to use medicine in a condition that is effective but without any harmful side-effects. There are a range of preparations such as infusions, decoctions, tinctures, extracts, tablets, pills, elixirs, electuaries, oils, with ointments and creams for external applications. The whole range of different parts of plants are used including roots, rhizomes, stems, barks, leaves, flowers, gums and oils.

Selection of the remedy depends upon the understanding and evaluation of an individual patient's temperament, the nature, severity and location of the disease. The physician also has to consider the sex, age, season, lifestyle, residence, occupation and previous treatment of the individual patient. Each of the above factors has to be applied in order to restore the lost or displaced equilibrium. An unbalanced organ provides an illustrative example. If the practitioner considers that an organ is diseased, then whilst paying attention to the other factors he has to select a single medicine with regard to the temperament of the organ affected, its structure, position and vitality.

Temperament is the energy pattern of the organ and provides information of the highest importance. When the original and normal energy pattern of the affected organ is known, it is relatively easy for the practitioner to assess the extent of abnormality and appropriate dosage and potency. If the affected organ is of hot temperament and the disease is cold, it indicates gross abnormality which will require strong, hot doses. However, if the original temperament is cold and the disease is also of the same quality then mild, cooling doses will re-establish the lost balance. The position and relationship of the affected organ is important too. Anatomical knowledge is helpful in the selection of the mode of administration of a remedy. The position of an organ can give an indication of the accessibility of an organ for remedial action. For example, the stomach is more easily influenced by mild medicament than the lungs. Each organ has interrelationships with other organs which help in determining treatment. The relationship of the liver to the kidneys and stomach is a useful example. If there is morbid matter in the upper part of the liver it can be easily eliminated through the kidneys, whereas if it is in the lower part of the liver it is better disposed of through the bowels. Correspondingly, the structure of an organ will give information which will indicate the level of penetration and absorption. Spongy organs respond differently to medicine from solid ones. The vitality of an organ is a significant factor in planning any treatment. The fundamental or vital organs such as the heart, brain and liver need milder medicine as any disturbance or too rapid change can cause serious complications. The vitality of an organ can also give an indication of the level of morbid matter and toxicity. Sensitivity and the normal function of the organ also have to be considered in the selection of a single remedy so as to avoid irritation or possible injurious effects.

Use of compound medicines

The use of compound medicaments is also employed in the treatment of internal diseases of complex and chronic nature. In traditional Islamic medicine, although the general preference is for the single remedy there are diseases in which using more than one substance combined in a coherent and thought-out basis enables a speedier cure. There are certain medicines which when used singly, even if in limited amounts have certain undesirable side-effects. Muslim practitioners developed this branch of the art and published authorative works known as *Aqrabadin* – 'Pharmacopeia'. The classical Greek and Indian sources were particularly utilized in the development of the use of compounds by Muslim physicians, and continue to be prepared and manufactured in the traditional methods by individual practitioners and natural medicine companies.[3] Works by masters of Islamic medicine such as Ibn Sina and Al-Razi's works continue to be used as basic references by today's practitioners. With the emergence of new stress deficiencies and patterns of disease there are formulations which take into account the new conditions. Generally, only the reputable *Hakims'* formulations are used. Usually the formulation or change in any traditional forms is a complicated process requiring a deep understanding of Materia Medica, and of human diseases, as well as considerable experience.

The use of the Qur'an in healing

An essential feature of the philosophy and practice of Islamic medicine is its harmony and ability to respond to the total needs of human beings. Islamic medicine has many facets which, on the one hand, relate to the physical needs and on the other hand are intimately bound with the higher order, and are responsive to the intangible aspects of the person. The whole phenomenon of creation is one that has the potential of uplifting and promoting creativity as well as the ability to degrade and debase. The existence and influence of destructive forces are also acknowledged, in particular the causes of insidious diseases of psycho-spiritual origin.

The Qur'an depicts this reality in vivid language in a number of places:

> Say: I seek refuge in the Lord of the Daybreak,
> From the evil of what he has created;
> From the evil of darkness when it gathers;
> From the evil of conjuring witches;
> From the evil of the envier when he envies.[4]

This awareness and understanding of the cosmological situation has enabled the *Hakims* to respond to diseases requiring intervention on a higher level. The Islamic *Shariha* – Divine Law – prohibits the practice and use of *Sihar* – magic – in treatment.[5] Muslim physicians use guidance and specific verses from the Qur'an in treatment. The Qur'an in its totality, and certain sections and verses in particular, is curative of serious conditions not amenable to other forms of treatment. The methods of using the Qur'an are many: *Tawiz* – literally meaning 'refuge' – in which sections of the Qur'an are used; *Dawah* – invocation – and *Ruqa*, are methods in which specific verses of the Qur'an are used in particular sequence and recited.[6]

Surgical intervention

Surgery has been an integral part of the practice and study of traditional Islamic medicine. Physicians were trained in both surgery and internal medicine. It was during Abu'l Qasim Al-Zahrawi's time that the practice of surgery reached its zenith. His classical work on the art. *Kitab Al-Tasrif* – 'The Book of Concession' – dealt with the subject in detail. Al-Zahrawi for the first time drew each instrument in colour. The general misunderstanding, namely that controlled dissection of the human body in the Islamic community prevents the growth and development of anatomical and physiological knowledge, is inaccurate. The study of human form has been an important aspect of Muslim scholarship to the extent that philosophers and mystics like Al-Ghazali thought it important in their gnostic traditions. Indeed, physicians and surgeons, for instance Ibn Al-Nafis, were aware of the lesser circulation in AH 687 (AD 1288).[7] Muslim surgeons used and developed a wide range of surgical instruments which were not only useful but beautiful and artistic in their looks. There were a number of surgical procedures that were used, from Caesarian section to complicated eye operations. The Muslim surgeon Thabit Ibn Qurra was using *Tanwim* – anaesthesia – in operations of the eyes as early as AH 850 (AD 1492).[8] The present situation in traditional Islamic medicine schools, unfortunately, does not reflect this outstanding surgical knowledge. Since colonial subjugation, in particular, the level of knowledge and skills of *Hakims* in surgery declined to such an extent that it may be said to be non-existent.[9]

CHAPTER 9

The future of Islamic medicine

Socio-cultural implications

In this final chapter, the focus will be to consider the future role of the Islamic health care tradition for health, well-being and its socio-cultural, economic and peace implications and benefits. Of course, these considerations do not constitute part of the accepted body of Islamic medical knowledge.

Given the prohibitive cost of technologically-based medicine, its inability to cure increasing chronic diseases, and the rising dissatisfaction – to the point of alienation – on the part of the intelligent public, a positive and important future is indicated for Islamic medicine.[1] The holistic and liberating paradigms, long clinical and therapeutic experiences, with a gentle, efficacious and rich treasury of natural medicaments, places Islamic medicine as the medicine of the future. It is surprising to what extent a tradition of health care with such positive characteristics as Islamic medicine has been hidden and ignored, and it would perhaps be helpful to consider why this has happened to such an economical and natural medicine.

The breakdown of Islamic culture was followed by subjugation and colonial domination. The colonial powers successfully disintegrated and fragmented most of the remaining Muslim societies. This physical disintegration was followed by the destruction of economic, political and socio-cultural and scientific structures. The traditional colleges of Islamic medicine, hospitals and professional organisations were systematically deprived of essential resources and freedom to practice and develop. The status and positive images of the *Hakims* and *Tabibs*, or physicians, were degraded. In a number of countries in the Muslim world their practices and teachings were made unlawful.[2]

However, the grassroots popularity of Islamic medicine and its appeal and practical usefulness, enabled it to be practised in various forms. The practice and teaching was well organised and deep-rooted in India, Bangladesh, Malaysia and Pakistan.[3] The political independence of Muslim lands has been accompanied by increasing awareness of cultural and scientific traditions and heritage. The Islamic reconstruction has also begun to give a prominence to Islamic sciences, including medicine.[4] The need for appropriate and effective medical care for masses of people provides new impetus for the future of Islamic medicine.

Economic considerations

Today, the practices of medicine is a major economical enterprise. The medical industry of our time is one of the largest and most powerful multi-nationals, particularly the pharmaceutical companies. The mechanistic approach of the dominant medical schools has led to a huge and cumbersome technological industry for diagnosis and treatment which knows no limits. Within the industrialised nations of Europe and the United States of America there is increasing dissatisfaction with high technology in medical matters which alienates the patients from their practitioners. The human dimension of care and sensitivity has been replaced by intrusive and insidious machines. The medical technology and pharmaceutical drugs sap away major chunks of the health care budget. The toxic side effects of drugs and most forms of mechanical diagnosis are becoming a health menace. Governments and research scholars are beginning to alert the public to the economically unsuitable health service and there is now serious re-assessment of the whole basis of health care.[5] Indeed, there is tremendous interest in, and growth of, human-oriented and economical health alternatives within most industrialised nations. Given these considerations it is important that non-industrialised nations maintain and develop traditional health care resources.

Implications for peace and happiness

The present age can be appropriately said to be the age of tranquillisers and violence. Each day some new tranquilliser is invented and introduced into the already extensive toxic armoury of chemical drugs, promising the ever-elusive state of peace and tranquillity. However, the range and level of mental and emotional disturbances and diseases are on the increase. The manifold stress of industrial life, a toxic environment and subversive, drug-based medicines compound the agony and suffering towards insanity and complete disintegration of the core of human beings. Highly mechanized hospitals with numerous specialists themselves appear to be victims of the process of de-humanisation by modern technocratic medicine. It is in this desperate context that Islamic medicine can provide the primordial wisdom, healing and creative energy with its gentle and effective treasury of natural medicine. The agonised and suffering masses could benefit enormously through the holistic and natural tradition of Islamic medicine. It is the benevolent creator who has created relief for mankind through His mercy and love. True health, peace and happiness comes through unification with the Truth.

Glossary

Aitidal: A dynamic condition of balance and equilibrium.

Akhlaat: The four primary biological fluids, blood, phlegm, bile and black bile. These constitute the biological basis of Islamic medicine.

Aql: An apprehending light, unique to human beings which guides the individual towards balanced decisions and actions.

Aqrabadin: A pharmacopoeia of compound medicines, giving details of individual substances and directions for their making and use.

Arrkan: The four basic elements, fire, air, water and earth.

Ayat: A Qur'anic term which means signs and manifestations which, when reflected upon, guide towards purpose and meaning.

Bayt Al-Hikmah: The House of Wisdom, an academy founded in Baghdad by the Abbasides to promote systematic research and development of sciences.

Bimaristan: a place for the sick, a hospital.

Bulghum: Phlegm, one of the four primary biological fluids, associated with water and being cold and moist in nature.

Diya: Blood money payable in respect of homicide.

93

Glossary

Deen-I-Fithra: The primordial tradition and way of life, Islam.

Ghaib: The hidden or unseen aspect of existence which is beyond normal human sensory perceptions.

Hakim: An individual endowed with knowledge, experience and wisdom, a sage. The title is given to a consultant physician of Islamic medicine.

Halal: Lawful and permitted food, nutrition and behaviour which is life-giving.

Hammam: A bath, generally deep cleansing, warm and cold alternating.

Haram: Opposite of *Halal*, unlawful, destructive nutrition or behaviour.

Hifz Al-Sihhah: Hygiene and public health matters with emphasis on prevention of ill-health.

Jism: The material body.

Khmar: Intoxicants, that which covers up the reason, alcohol.

Latif: Subtle and penetrative force.

Miswak: A traditional root used from the time of Muhammad, P.B.U.H., for cleansing of the teeth and mouth.

Muffradat: Individual drugs, usually of plant origin, in their natural states. Class of Islamic medical literature which deals with the study and uses of natural substances.

Murakkabat: Compound medicines, prepared from a number of individual substances. A class of Islamic medical texts dealing with use and making of compound medicines.

Mizaj: A dynamic functional state which reflects the energy pattern of an individual person or a thing.

Nafs: The self, which can have a number of states: *Ammara*, fossilized and insensitive; *Lawwama*, reproachful and agitated; *Mutmainna*, tranquil or

94

balanced state.

Qalb: A non-material principle which regulates the predominantly psycho-emotional life of a person.

Reeh: A harmful type of gaseous wind, usually in the stomach.

Rooh: The vital force. A purposeful and dynamic force that permeates the human organism. Muslim physicians give different names to it depending on its function and location: *Hawania*, centred in the heart and maintains life; *Nafsania*, located in the brain and promotes sensation and movement; *Tabayya*, located in the liver for preservation of the individual and in the ovaries and testicles for the preservation of the species.

Ruh: The spirit which is of divine origin and is transcendental.

Safra: Yellow bile, one of the four primary biological fluids, corresponding to the element of fire and hot and dry in Nature.

Sakoon: A state of peace and tranquillity; the result of unification with the truth.

Sauda: Black bile, one of the four primary biological fluids, corresponding to the earth and being cold and dry.

Sharih: A path, paradigm of principles and practices which enables human beings to live in harmony with reality.

Taharah: Purity and cleanliness of an individual and community.

Taqwa: A state and consciousness which guides one to refrain from destructive behaviour.

Tibb: Literal meaning 'Nature' refers to holistic medicine; *Tibb I Nabwai* – prophetic medicine.

Wahi: Revelation, that is, direct knowledge from the creator.

Glossary

Zahir: The external or outward aspects of creation and existence.

Notes and references

1 Historical background

1. T.P. Hughes, *Dictionary of Islam*, Cosmos Publications, New Delhi, 1978, p. 17.

2. N. Groom, *Frankincense and Myrrh*, Longman, London, 1981, p. 96.

3. Hughes, op. cit., p. 18.

4. The Qur'an, 53:19-20. The Qur'anic references are quoted in this format, which refers to the chapter or *Sura*, as it is known in Arabic, followed by the number of the *Ayat* – verse or sentence.

5. A.A. Maududi, *The Philosophy of Hajj*, Idra Tar-Juman-ul-Quran, Lahore, 1976, p. 20.

6. S. Qutb, *In the Shade of the Qur'an*, Muslim Welfare House London Publishers, London, 1979, p. 66.

7. M.B. Badri, *Islam and Alcoholism*, American Trust Publications, London, 1978, p. 11.

8. Ibid., p. 11.

9. Ibid., p. 9.

10. Ibid., p. 12.

11. M. Ullmann, *Islamic Medicine*, Edinburgh University Press, 1978, p. 1.

12. The Qur'an, 96:1-5.

13. The Qur'an, 16:58-59.

14. The Qur'an, 4:22.

Notes and references

15. Al-Suyuti, Tibb-Ul-Nabbi, *Osiris*, 1962, Vol. 4, p. 51.

16. S.H.H. Nadvi, *Medical Philosophy in Islam and the Contribution of Muslims in the Advancement of Medical Sciences*, Academia, University of Durban, Durban, 1983, p. 7.

17. C. Elgood, *A Medical History of Persia and the Eastern Caliphate*, Cambridge University Press, 1951, p. 49.

18. Ibid., p. 49.

19. E.G. Browne, *Arabian Medicine*, Cambridge University Press, 1962, p. 15.

20. M.Z. Siddiqi, *Studies in Arabic and Persian Medical Literature*, Calcutta University, 1959, p. 24.

21. S.H. Nasr, *Islamic Science*, World of Islam Festival Publishing Co., London, 1976, p. 187.

22. Ibid., p. 189.

23. Elgood, op. cit., p. 70.

24. Ibid., p. 76.

25. Ibid., p. 175.

26. M.H. Shah, *The General Principles of Avicennas Canon of Medicine*, Naveed Clinic, Karachi, 1966, p. 439.

27. Nasr, op. cit., p. 187.

28. S.H. Nasr, *Science and Civilization in Islam*, Harvard University Press, 1968, p. 213.

29. M. Said, *Hamdard Medical Digest*, 1959, Vol. 1-2, p. 136.

30. Personal communication and discussion with *Hakim* Muhammad Nabi Khan and *Hakim* Muhammad Riaz Qersih Sahib.

2 Philosophical concepts

1. The essential philosophical concepts are derived from the Qur'an, *The Hadith* – 'Traditions and Sayings of the Prophet, P.B.U.H.', and the works of Islamic scholars such as Al-Ghazali and Ibn Arabi.

Notes and references

2. S.H. Hasr, *An Introduction to Islamic Cosmological Doctrines*, Thames and Hudson, London, 1978, pp. 101-2.
3. The Qur'an 23: 12-14.
4. Ibn Sina, *The General Principles of Medicine*, Naveed Clinic, Karachi, 1966, p. 142.
5. S.H. Nasr, *Science and Civilization in Islam*, Harvard University Press, 1968, p. 184.

3 Psychological foundation

1. Al-Ghazali, *Kimya-I-Sadat*, Sheikh Ghulam Ali and Sons Publishers, Lahore, 1977, p. 60.
2. The Qur'an 89: 27.
3. The Qur'an 75: 2.
4. The Qur'an 12: 53.
5. Ibn Sina, *Kitab-Ul-Adwiya Qalbiya*, Iran Society, Calcutta, 1956, p. 1.

4 Physiological basis

1. *Quwa* – energy is a central concept in Islamic medicine.
2. O.C. Gruner, *The Canon of Medicine of Avicenna*, Augustus M. Kelley, New York, 1970, p. 34.
3. Ibid., p. 35.
4. The Qur'an, 76:5.
5. This is the classical way of studying anatomy and physiology.

5 Pathogenesis

1. One can see the holistic nature of Islamic medicine, in that it takes account of the multifarious factors acting and reacting upon an individual.
2. M.H. Shah, *The General Principles of Avicennas Canon of Medicine*, Naveed Clinic, Karachi, 1966, p. 156.
3. The water of Zam Zam occupies a special curative

and preventative place in Islamic medicine. One of the characteristics of Zam Zam is that it is not subjective to putrefaction like other waters.

4. The preventative measures can be rightly referred to as ecological adaptation. The modern speciality of clinical ecology is a re-discovery of the wider principles illustrated in this chapter. See R. Mackarness, *Chemical Victims*, Pan, London, 1980, pp. 1-20.

6 *Diagnosis*

1. These are the indicators of health and balance, see O.C. Gruner, *The Canon of Medicine of Avicenna*, Augustus M. Kelley, New York, 1970, pp. 381-456.

2. The central clinical concept in Islamic Medicine is that of *Mizaj* – temperament, evaluation of energy patterns.

3. I am grateful to *Hakim* Noor Muhammad Hani for his help in the study of pulse diagnosis.

4. Gruner, op. cit., pp. 323-46.

5. Ibid., p. 355.

7 *Preventative aspects of Islamic medicine*

1. The Latin name of the particular tree is *Salvadora Persica*, whose preventative and curative value has been studied analytically in Switzerland by Pharba Basle Ltd.

2. Al-Ghazali, *Kimya-I-Sadat*, Sheikh Ghulam Ali & Sons, Lahore, 1977, pp. 164-83.

3. Ibid., p. 231.

4. Bukhri, *Sahih Al Bukari*, Vol. 7, Dar-Ul-Fikar, Makkha, pp. 418-20.

5. The Qur'an 2:222.

6. The *shariha* and traditions of the prophet Muhammad, P.B.U.H. specifically advised these categories not to fast.

Notes and references

8 Principles of treatment

1. This is a classical division of Materia Medica by Muslim physicians and scholars.

2. The research in our own age is also moving towards this realization that human beings contain the physio-chemical constituents of the earth as well as the different forces.

3. Dawakhna Hakim Ajmal Khan Ltd. of Lahore, *Methods of Medicament Preparations*.

4. The Qur'an, 113: 1-5.

5. The Qur'an, 20:69.

6. A. Ali, *Amal-I-Qurani*, Naz Publishing House, Delhi, p. 15.

7. S.H. Nasr, *Science and Civilization in Islam*, Harvard University Press, 1969, p. 213.

8. M. Bayrakdar, 'The First Use of Anaesthesia', *Imam*, 1984, pp. 52-3.

9. The reasons are many for this situation, with the most apparent being that the government is reluctant to fund surgery in traditional colleges as well as the Muslim physicians' own lack of surgical skills.

9 Future of Islamic medicine

1. S. Fulder and R. Monr, *The Status of Complementary Medicine*, The Threshold Foundation, London, 1981, pp. 1-19. This and many other reports and publications indicate the need for holistic health care.

2. In parts of the Arabian Peninsula even today *Hakims* are not allowed to practice or set up professional organisations.

3. Pakistan is one of the leading pioneers in promoting Islamic medicine with central and regional government funding. The government regulates the teaching and research through a national council of *Tibb* based in Islamabad and regulated by Act of Parliament.

101

Notes and references

4. The Islamic Medicine Organization (I.M.O.) in Kuwait is an example as well as the work of *Hakim* Mohd Said, President of Hamdard Foundation, Karachi, Pakistan. See also Z. Sardar, *Science and Technology in the Middle East*, Longman, London, 1982, pp. 18-23.
5. I. Kennedy, *The Unmasking of Medicine*, George Allen & Unwin, London, 1981, pp. 117-69.

Index

Index

Index

Index